DEH313
Social Sciences/School of Education/Institute of Educational Technology
An Interfaculty Third Level Course

PRINCIPLES OF SOCIAL AND EDUCATIONAL RESEARCH

BLOCK 4

UNIT 17/18
ANALYSIS OF UNSTRUCTURED DATA
David Boulton and Martyn Hammersley

UNIT 19/20
ANALYSIS OF STRUCTURED DATA
Judith Calder

UNIT 21
CRITICAL ANALYSIS OF TEXT
Victor Jupp

The Open University

DEH313 Course Team

Roger Sapsford, Senior Lecturer in Research Methods, Faculty of Social Sciences, and Course Team Chair

Michele Aylard, Course Secretary, Psychology

Andrew Bertie, Academic Computing Services

Judith Calder, Deputy Director, Institute of Educational Technology

Tim Clark, Research Fellow, School of Management

Jack Clegg, Producer, Audio-visual Services

Stephen Clift, Editor, Social Sciences

Sarah Crompton, Graphic Designer

Ruth Finnegan, Professor in Comparative Social Institutions, Faculty of Social Sciences

Adam Gawronski, Academic Computing Services

Martyn Hammersley, Reader in Educational and Social Research, School of Education

Fiona Harris, Editor, Social Sciences

Kevin McConway, Senior Lecturer in Statistics, Faculty of Mathematics

Ann Macfarlane, Secretary, School of Education

Sheila Peace, Lecturer, Department of Health and Social Welfare, Institute of Health, Welfare and Community Education

David Scott-Macnab, Editor, Social Sciences

Paul Smith, Media Librarian

Keith Stribley, Course Manager, Faculty of Social Sciences

Betty Swift, Lecturer in Research Methods, Institute of Educational Technology

Ray Thomas, Senior Lecturer in Applied Social Sciences, Faculty of Social Sciences

Pat Vasiliou, Discipline Secretary, Psychology

Steve Wilkinson, Producer, BBC

Michael Wilson, Senior Lecturer in Social Sciences, Faculty of Social Sciences

Consultant Authors

Pamela Abbott, Principal Lecturer in Sociology and Social Policy, University of Plymouth

David Boulton, Lecturer, Faculty of Community Studies and Education, Manchester Polytechnic

Peter Foster, Senior Lecturer in Education, Crewe and Alsager College of Higher Education

Victor Jupp, Principal Lecturer in Sociology, Polytechnic of Newcastle upon Tyne

William Schofield, Lecturer, Department of Experimental Psychology, University of Cambridge

External Assessor

Robert Burgess, Professor of Sociology, University of Warwick

Advisory Panel

Peter Aggleton, Senior Lecturer in Policy and Management in Education, Goldsmiths' College, University of London

Jeanette James, Consultant Psychologist and Open University Tutor

Elizabeth Murphy, Research Fellow, University of Nottingham

The Open University
Walton Hall, Milton Keynes
MK7 6AA

First published 1993

Copyright © 1993 The Open University

All rights reserved. No part of this publication may be reproduced, stored in a retrieval system or transmitted, in any form or by any means, without written permission from the publisher or a licence from the Copyright Licensing Agency Limited. Details of such licences (for reprographic reproduction) may be obtained from the Copyright Licensing Agency Ltd of 90 Tottenham Court Road, London WC1P 9HE.

Edited, designed and typeset by the Open University

Printed in the United Kingdom by the Alden Press, Oxford

ISBN 0 7492 0156 8

This text forms part of an Open University Third Level Course. If you would like a copy of *Studying with the Open University*, please write to the Central Enquiry Service, P.O. Box 200, The Open University, Walton Hall, Milton Keynes MK7 6YZ, United Kingdom. If you have not already enrolled on the course and would like to buy this or other Open University material, please write to Open University Educational Enterprises Ltd, 12 Cofferidge Close, Stony Stratford, Milton Keynes MK11 1BY, United Kingdom.

1.1

4462/deh313b4u17/18i1.1

UNIT 17/18 ANALYSIS OF UNSTRUCTURED DATA

Prepared for the Course Team by David Boulton and Martyn Hammersley

CONTENTS

Associated study materials		4
1	**Introduction**	5
2	**The complementary perspectives of reader and researcher**	7
3	**Types of qualitative data analysis**	8
4	**The process of analysis**	10
	4.1 Data preparation	10
	4.2 Starting the analysis	14
5	**An example**	18
6	**Reflexivity and the assessment of validity**	22
7	**Conclusion**	23
Further reading		23
References		24
Acknowledgements		25
Appendix 1		26
Appendix 2		36

ASSOCIATED STUDY MATERIALS

Reader, Chapter 3, 'Qualitative research and psychological theorizing', by K.L. Henwood and N.F. Pidgeon.

Offprints Booklet 4, 'The ethnographic study of cognitive systems', by C.O. Frake.

Offprints Booklet 4, 'Streetcorner encounters', by M. Punch.

Audio-Cassette 1.

Data disk 'DATASET: LYNN.SW2'

1 INTRODUCTION

In this unit we shall look at some of the problems involved and techniques used in analysing unstructured data. This kind of data is central to qualitative research. Indeed, 'qualitative data' and 'unstructured data' are often treated as synonyms, though unstructured data are also used outside of qualitative research. (You may remember that, in Unit 14, Betty Swift outlined some of the ways in which survey researchers handle such data.) We shall concentrate here on the strategies used by qualitative researchers, but this does not imply any sharp distinction between quantitative and qualitative forms of analysis.

What we mean by 'unstructured data' is data that are not already coded in terms of the researcher's analytical categories. Such data consist mainly, but not exclusively, of written texts of various sorts: published and unpublished documents (including official government reports, personal diaries, letters, minutes of meetings, etc.), as well as field note descriptions written by researchers, transcripts of audio- or video-recordings, and so on. These kinds of data contrast with structured data, which include, for example, tallies recording respondents' choices from pre-specified answers or the observed frequencies of various predefined sorts of activity. The structuring of data can take two forms:

1. It may result from the physical control of responses, as in experiments or structured questionnaires, where people are effectively forced to choose one or other response by the researcher.

2. It may be produced by the application of a set of categories to 'unconstrained' behaviour, as in the case of systematic observation or the coding of free responses to questionnaire items in terms of a pre-established coding scheme.

What is distinctive about unstructured data is that they involve neither of these forms of structuring.

It is important not to be misled by the term 'unstructured', however. It does not mean that the data lack *all* structure. All data are structured in some ways. For instance, written documents will display lexical, grammatical and semantic structuring; and, more significantly, they will also be structured by the concerns and intentions of the writer. Furthermore, where these texts describe events of various kinds, those events will themselves have some sort of structure which the texts capture more or less accurately. These various types of structure will often be of interest to analysts. For instance, when we analyse documents we usually want to know how they were shaped by the writer's intended audience, since this may well affect what inferences we can reasonably draw from what is written. Equally, we will often want to try to find out how what the document says relates to the patterns of events it describes.

It is also necessary to remember that to say that data are unstructured does not mean that they are uninfluenced by the researcher. Even documents written in the past for purposes completely unrelated to research become part of a corpus of research data only through a process of search and/or selection by the researcher (and perhaps also of negotiation by the researcher with those who control access to the relevant documents). Furthermore, when the data are observational field notes, we must add the possibility of reactivity, of how the researcher may have affected what was observed (see Unit 12, in particular Section 2), as well as how he or she decided to select and describe what is portrayed. With interview data it is also necessary to remember that the questions asked are likely to have influenced the answers given, to one degree or another and in one way or another. To say that data are unstructured does not imply, then, that they are unaffected by the researcher; and the effect of the researcher on the data is an important consideration we must bear in mind in the course of data analysis, as well as when reading the results of data analysis done by others. This is true whatever form of research is involved.

There has been much argument about the relative value of unstructured and structured data. At one time, under the influence of some versions of the scientific model (see Unit 1/2), most social researchers believed that structured data were superior (indeed perhaps that they were the only legitimate form of data). This belief was founded on the assumption that this type of data facilitates precise and replicable measurements of people's behaviour, and that such measurement is essential if scientific hypotheses are to be subjected to effective test. Some researchers still believe this, and most researchers recognize that structured data can be of value for certain purposes. However, there has been a strong trend over the past few decades, in many fields of research, towards the increasing use of unstructured data, as part of a general shift towards qualitative research.

This shift has arisen in part from criticism of much research relying on structured data for ignoring sources of potential error built into those data. Indeed, it has been recognized that the very process of structuring data can introduce error. Physical structuring of data of the kind involved in experimental research is likely to increase reactivity, and especially procedural reactivity. In other words, people's behaviour will be influenced by their awareness that they are taking part in an experiment, and this may make their responses unrepresentative of their behaviour in non-experimental situations (see, for example, Wuebben *et al.*, 1974). Post-structuring of data of the sort used in systematic observation, on the other hand, is often criticized for involving arbitrary decisions that force events into categories which they do not fit (Delamont and Hamilton, 1984; see also McIntyre and Macleod, 1978). These dangers are recognized by quantitative researchers, but are generally regarded as controllable by good design of experimental procedures or by careful framing and piloting of questionnaires and observational schedules. However, the critics have taken these problems to be more fundamental, sometimes even regarding structured data as always by their very nature an arbitrary construction on the part of researchers, one that bears little or no relationship to the reality that it is supposed to document. As is often the case, the truth probably lies somewhere between these two contrasting views.

These different views about structured and unstructured data reflect, of course, more than just disagreements about the specific issues mentioned above. They form part of the broader debates about the purposes and proper nature of social research that were discussed in Unit 1/2.

READING

From the Reader, you should now read Chapter 3, 'Qualitative research and psychological theorizing', by Karen L. Henwood and Nick F. Pidgeon. In this article the authors outline the main lines of the debates about quantitative and qualitative research, with particular reference to psychology, a field where qualitative approaches are still less influential than quantitative method. They also provide a useful overview of the sort of qualitative data analysis we shall be primarily concerned with in this unit. As you read their article, make a note of the main features of what they refer to as 'grounded theory'.

Henwood and Pidgeon present qualitative research as based on an epistemological paradigm that is distinct from that of quantitative research. At the same time, they note that the two paradigms share something in common and that, in practice, methods are selected on grounds additional to epistemological considerations. Furthermore, they emphasize that the two paradigms are not incommensurable: it is possible to engage in fruitful debate about their various assumptions.

Our view is broadly similar. While we recognize that qualitative research is often associated with methodological and epistemological arguments that are different from those espoused by most quantitative methodologists, and while we accept the value of some of those assumptions, we do not think it is helpful to see qualitative and quantitative research as based on clearly distinct and incompatible paradigms. Thus, we do not regard the use of structured and unstructured data as representing a commitment on the part of researchers to different research paradigms. We view both sorts of data as having varying advantages and disadvantages for particular research purposes. Which should be used depends in large part on the goals of the research, and the circumstances in which these are to be pursued; and often the two sorts of data may need to be combined. It should be noted, though, that this is by no means the only or even the predominant view about this issue among social scientists. There is much disagreement, even amongst qualitative researchers, about what the relationship is or should be between qualitative and quantitative research (see, for example, Smith and Heshusius, 1986; Bryman, 1988; Walker and Evers, 1988; Hammersley, 1992, ch. 9).

2 THE COMPLEMENTARY PERSPECTIVES OF READER AND RESEARCHER

Unit 3/4 looked at how to begin assessing the validity of the claims and evidence found in research reports, and many of the examples used there involved unstructured data. It was suggested that in such assessments two considerations are important:

1 Plausibility: the extent to which a claim seems likely to be true given its relationship to what we and others currently take to be knowledge that is beyond reasonable doubt.

2 Credibility: whether the claim is of a kind that, given what we know about how the research was carried out, we can judge it to be very likely to be true.

Where a claim is neither sufficiently plausible nor credible to be accepted, it was suggested, we must look at the evidence offered in support of it (if there is any). And when we do so we must be concerned with the plausibility and credibility of the evidence itself and the strength of its relationship to the claim it is intended to support.

In assessing the plausibility and credibility of the claims and evidence presented in a research report, in effect we are engaging in a dialogue with the writer of that report. Of course, it is a dialogue in which one side (that of the researcher) is only imagined by the reader, although on some occasions it may turn into a real dialogue: for example, in the case of a book review to which the author replies.

It is important to recognize that a similar dialogue, again with one side largely imaginary, takes place in doing research. In framing research questions, selecting cases, gathering and interpreting data, the researcher constantly has an audience, indeed perhaps several audiences, in mind. So, in the course of their work, researchers continually ask themselves whether their interpretations of data are sufficiently plausible and credible, what other data may be necessary to check and support these interpretations, etc. And their answers to these questions will be shaped by their anticipations of how particular sorts of audience will react to their interpretations.

Of course, there is an important difference between the dialogues in which readers and researchers engage. Whereas the reader starts with the main claims presented by an author and, as and when necessary, moves to what evidence is given in support of them, the researcher on the other hand begins with data (and, of course, with a lot more than is ever likely to appear in the research report) and must move, somehow, from those data to some major claims. However, despite coming from different ends, as it were, the analytical work of reader and researcher is similar in character. To some degree, in order to understand a piece of research one has to reconstruct the activity of the researcher, to imagine what he or she was trying to do and how that task was tackled; though, of course, how far this is possible will depend on the information available about the research process.

In this unit we shall look in some detail at the process of analysing unstructured data. This should enable you to get a clearer sense of what is involved in qualitative data analysis and also, perhaps, make more effective the dialogue you engage in when you read texts employing this sort of analysis.

3 TYPES OF QUALITATIVE DATA ANALYSIS

There is considerable diversity within qualitative research in approaches to data analysis. One major source of variation is the character of the intended product. Unit 3/4 identified several different types of argument that were to be found in research reports: definitions, descriptions, explanations, predictions, evaluations, prescriptions and theories. All of these, with the exception of definitions, can also be *end-products* of research. Thus, some research is largely descriptive in character: for example, involving the production of a narrative account of some series of events. It is rare for a whole research report to take this form, but there are some examples that come close to this. A striking one is Susan Krieger's account of the life of a radio station. Here is her summary of the study:

> The study was begun in 1972 and consisted of eleven months of interviewing persons involved with the station, obtaining documentary evidence from them and from other sources, visiting the station, and listening to it. The next two years were spent in writing a text which described a process of cooptation in the life of the station over the years 1967–72. The station had been closely associated with the Summer of Love in San Francisco in 1967. It was thought to have been the first hard rock 'hippy' radio station in the country. In the five years since, it had become increasingly commercial, professional, and successful, and was frequently criticized for having sold out to the establishment.
>
> (Krieger, 1979, pp.167–8)

Sometimes qualitative research produces narratives which document the course of the research project itself, rather than a sequence of events independent of the researcher. An interesting journalistic example of this is John Cornwell's book on the death of Pope John Paul I (Cornwell, 1990). Here is how his book starts:

> On a morning late in October 1987 I set out for the Vatican from a hotel on the Via Vitelleschi close to the Castel Sant' Angelo. It was warm for the time of year and I felt exhilarated as I turned from a side street to view the grandeur of Saint Peter's Basilica in misty sunlight from the Via della Conciliazone, the ceremonial route that sweeps grandly from the Tiber to Saint Peter's Square. The tourists had mostly departed and the pavements were empty except for those familiar figures of Catholic officialdom, the Roman clergy. Square-shaped, wearing black cassocks and raincoats, thick-soled shoes, black berets, bespectacled, they moved impassively, separately, yet all at the same dogged pace towards their destination, the Vatican City. To the children of Rome they are known as *bagarozzi* — black beetles.

I began to walk in the same direction as the priests, towards the smallest state in the world, and perhaps the most secretive.

My appointment was with one Archbishop John Foley, President of the Commission for Social Communications, an official Vatican media and public-relations office. I had been instructed by his secretary to report at the gate known as the Arco delle Campane, on the left of Saint Peter's Basilica. One of the two Swiss Guards beneath the arch stood with halberd presented as the other approached me: his gingery hair shorn to the skull, wide in his bulky cloak. He saluted and waited for me to speak, solidly barring my way. On telling him the nature of my errand, he cried out gutturally, 'Permissions office!' and waved me through the gate and to the left of the archway.

(Cornwell, 1990, p.3)

Almost the whole of Cornwell's book takes this narrative form. This is very rare in social research, but it is not uncommon to find stretches of narrative commentary reporting the experiences of the researcher. (You may remember that Maurice Punch's article 'Observation and the police', which you read for Unit 12, begins in this way.) Furthermore, it is quite common these days to find so-called 'reflexive accounts' or 'natural histories' of particular studies written by researchers. One of the first and best known is Whyte's account of his research on various aspects of the Italian-American community of Boston's North End in the 1940s (Whyte, 1981; see also Boelen, 1992; Whyte, 1992). Such reflexive accounts of the research process may, of course, be an important source of information relevant to the assessment of studies' findings. (You will find lists of reflexive accounts of research in Hammersley and Atkinson, 1983, and in Walford, 1987.)

There are other sorts of largely descriptive research. Some is focused on the way in which discourse (verbal interaction or written text) is patterned (see Potter and Wetherell, 1987). Discourse analysis is becoming increasingly common in sociology and social psychology, and in other areas too, and it takes a variety of forms. It may be concerned with mundane features of everyday life; for example, with the way that turn-taking is organized in conversations. Other work is concerned with presuppositions built into what is said or written by some individual or group. For example, Schegloff (1971) looks in detail at the process of giving directions to those unable to find their way. He notes how the character of the directions given is context-sensitive: it is affected, for instance, by the location in which the directions are being given and by the geographical knowledge that the recipient is assumed already to have. Other discourse analytical work focuses on more controversial areas. Thus, Billig (1991) has looked at the way that different 'ideologies' come into conflict in discourse surrounding, for example, medicine and social work.

Another distinctive form of largely descriptive qualitative research, this time in cultural anthropology, is devoted to documenting the array of concepts used by a particular group to deal with some aspect of their experience. This approach is sometimes referred to as ethnosemantics.

READING

You should now read 'The ethnographic study of cognitive systems', by C.O. Frake, which is reproduced in Offprints Booklet 4. In this article, Frake provides an outline and illustration of the characteristic approach of ethnosemantic investigation.

Ethnosemantics is directed towards producing a detailed account of the array of concepts used by a particular group of people to make sense of their environment. Much qualitative research takes this as part of its focus: qualitative researchers often place great emphasis on the importance of understanding the perspectives of the people they are studying. However, normally they seek to do this simply by listening for the categories that people use in informal talk or interviews, rather than by using the rather more structured elicitation devices favoured by ethnosemanticists. Equally important, they generally do not restrict themselves to description of people's perspectives, being also concerned with the causes and consequences of these. And, often, they do not draw a sharp distinction between description, explanation, and theory development, so that much qualitative research seems to be aimed at producing all three kinds of product simultaneously (Hammersley, 1992, ch. 1).

READING

At this point, you should read the article 'Streetcorner encounters', by Maurice Punch, which is to be found in Offprints Booklet 4. This comes from the same book as the reflexive account of this research by Punch which you read for Unit 12. It will give you a sense of the kind of product that much qualitative research generates, combining description, explanation and theory.

4 THE PROCESS OF ANALYSIS

In this section we shall look at what is actually involved in doing qualitative analysis, focusing on what is the most commonly used set of procedures, often referred to as grounded theorizing, which was discussed by Henwood and Pidgeon in the article you read earlier. A common concern in qualitative data analysis, and especially in grounded theorizing, is the identification of the perspectives of various groups of people involved in a setting, the documentation of the problems that they face in their lives, and the description of the strategies that they have developed to deal with those problems. This provides a general framework for the analysis, but the substance must come from the data.

4.1 DATA PREPARATION

Of course, data are rarely obtained in an immediately analysable form — usually they must be prepared before analysis can begin. The need for data preparation is most obvious with audio- and video-recordings. While listening to or watching a recording is a good way to familiarize oneself with the data, for the purposes of analysis it is usually necessary to transcribe recordings, or at least to produce a summary and index of what is on them; a task which is, of course, quite time consuming.

ACTIVITY 1

Audio-cassette 1, Side 1, begins with an introduction by Roger Sapsford which is followed by a recording of an interview between Senga Bond and Lynn Sadler, a sister on a medical ward in North Tees Hospital. You will be carrying out an analysis of this interview later. Here we want you to transcribe the opening section of the interview, down to where Senga asks Lynn to describe a patient when she or he is poorly. Do this now.

Please do *not* look at the transcript contained in the Audio-Visual Handbook before doing this. Once you have finished transcription of this section, however, look at the transcript in the Handbook and compare it with yours. Identify the divergences and think about why they have occurred.

You will have probably found yourself faced with some difficult decisions in making this transcription. For one thing, you might have wondered about how best to set out your transcription of what each speaker said. Also, you will have noticed that people do not always talk one at a time, even in one-to-one interaction, so that often the talk overlaps. As a result, the question arises: does one transcribe the talk as if only one person were talking at any one time, or, on the other hand, try to represent overlaps where they occur? You will find that the transcript in the Audio-Visual Handbook adopts the former strategy. Again, you will have discovered that people do not talk in sentences. They sometimes break off and restart what they are saying, they pause in the middle of what might otherwise seem to be a sentence, and do not always pause at what seems like the end of a sentence. Also, in an interview there are a lot of 'ums' and 'uhrs', some of them coming from the person listening, and we need to decide whether these should be transcribed. In all of these respects, and others, you may have found that your transcription differed from ours.

There is a variety of conventions in terms of which audio-recordings can be transcribed — and which set of conventions is appropriate depends partly on the purposes of the research. For example, where detailed analysis of the process of discourse will be involved, pauses may need to be timed, overlaps in talk between one speaker and another clearly marked, etc., as well as other verbal (and perhaps even non-verbal) features of the talk included. You may remember a quite detailed transcription scheme being used in the article 'Gender imbalances in the primary classroom' by Jane and Peter French, which you read in Block 1. (Look back at this now.) By contrast, the transcripts normally used by qualitative researchers who are not so closely concerned with discourse features contain much less detail and are often imprecise in the linguistic sense, as is the case with our transcript of the interview between Senga and Lynn.

How detailed a transcription needs to be, and what does and does not need to be included, then, are matters of judgement that depend on the purposes of the research (see Ochs, 1979). But the form of transcription will also partly depend, of course, on the amount of information that a recording supplies. Obviously, video-recordings supply much more information than audio-recordings, and special forms of transcription have been developed for handling these (see, for example, Goodwin, 1981). Also important is the quality of the recording, and this will depend on the nature of what is recorded as well as on the recording equipment. Clearly, in the case of an audio-recording the more speakers involved, and the more background noise, the more difficult it is to get adequate recording quality. Similarly, with video-recordings the more crowded the setting, and the more movement there is, the more difficult it may be to see what is going on.

In assessing a study that draws on transcriptions and provides a transcription scheme, a useful question to ask, therefore, is whether the scheme used is appropriate, given the sort of data collected and the purposes of the research. Does it include all the relevant information that seems likely to have been available, given the nature of the recordings? On the other hand, does it provide too much detail, thereby making it more difficult to assess the evidential status of the data presented in the report? Does it seem likely to be accurate in the relevant respects?

The need for the preparation of data is not restricted to audio- and video-recordings. Field notes are often written initially in jotted form and then written out, and filled in, later. (You may remember that the feedback given to Activity 11 in Unit 12 provided an example of jotted and filled out field notes.) There are variations in format and style between researchers in the writing of field notes, just as there are in the transcription of audio- and video-recordings. In general, though, the aim is to make the notes as concrete as possible, minimizing the amount of questionable inference involved. The following quotation from Hammersley and Atkinson (1983) illustrates this point:

> Below we reproduce two extracts from notes that purport to recapture the same interaction. They are recognizably 'about' the same people and the same events. By the same token, neither lays any claim to completeness. The first obviously compresses things to an extreme extent, and the

second summarizes some things, and explicitly acknowledges that some parts of the conversation are missing altogether:

'1. The teacher told his colleagues in the staffroom about the wonders of a progressive school he had been to visit the day before. He was attacked from all sides. As I walked up with him to his classroom he continued talking of how the behaviour of the pupils at X had been marvellous. We reached his room. I waited outside, having decided to watch what happened in the hall in the build up to the morning assembly. He went into his classroom and immediately began shouting at his class. He was taking it out on them for not being like the pupils at X.

2. (Walker gives an enthusiastic account of X to his colleagues in the staffroom. There is an aggressive reaction.)

GREAVES: Projects are not education, just cutting out things.

WALKER: Oh no, they don't allow that, there's a strict check on progress.

HOLTON: The more I hear of this the more wishy-washy it sounds.

(…)

WALKER There's a craft resources area and pupils go and do some dress-making or woodwork when they want to, when it fits into their project.

HOLTON: You need six weeks' basic teaching in woodwork or metalwork.

(…)

HOLTON: How can an immature child of that age do a project?

WALKER: Those children were self-controlled and well-behaved.

(…)

HOLTON: Sounds like utopia.
DIXON: Gimmicky.
WALKER: There's no vandalism. They've had the books four years and they've been used a lot and I could see the pupils were using them, but they looked new, the teacher had told them that if they damaged the books she would have to replace them herself.

(…)

HOLTON: Sounds like those kids don't need teaching.

((Walker and I go up to his room: he continues his praise for X. When we reach his room I wait outside to watch the hall as the build up for the morning assembly begins. He enters his room and immediately begins shouting. The thought crosses my mind that the contrast between the pupils at X he has been describing and defending to his colleagues and the "behaviour" of his own pupils may be a reason for his shouting at the class, but, of course, I don't know what was going on in the classroom.))

(( )) = observer descriptions.

(…) = omission of parts of conversation in record.'

(Hammersley 1980)

The second version is much more concrete in its treatment of the events; indeed, much of the time the speech of the actors themselves is preserved. We can inspect the notes with a fair assurance that we are gaining information on how the participants themselves described things, who said what to whom, and so on. When we compress and summarize we do not simply lose 'interesting' detail and 'local colour', we lose vital information.

(Hammersley and Atkinson, 1983, pp.152–3)

This emphasis on concrete description in field notes does not mean, of course, that researchers are uninterested in how the events they observe and record in their field notes might be interpreted. Indeed, any interpretations that the researcher thinks of in the course of observation or while writing up the field notes are usually noted. But care is taken to avoid those interpretations structuring the data recording itself, since they may turn out to be wrong. And, usually, such interpretations are distinguished typographically from the field notes proper; for example, by being put into brackets.

Also included in field notes may be the researcher's personal feelings about what has been observed or about her or his own role. Once again, these will usually be recorded in a way that marks them off from the observational record. Apart from its value in indicating possible sources of bias in the data, reflection by the researcher on her or his own experience in the setting may also facilitate the process of understanding the people being studied. Bogdan and Taylor illustrate this from their studies of a hospital for people with learning difficulties (the 'state institution') and a job training agency:

> What you feel may be what your subjects feel or may have felt in the past. Your first impressions may be the same ones that others have had. You should use your feelings, beliefs, preconceptions, and prejudices to help you develop hypotheses. The following comments are excerpted from field-notes in the state institution study.
>
>> I feel quite bored and depressed on the ward tonight. I wonder if this has anything to do with the fact that there are only two attendants working now. With only two attendants on, there are fewer diversions and less bantering. Perhaps this is why the attendants always complain about there not being enough of them. After all, there is never more work here than enough to occupy two attendants' time so it's not the fact that they can't get their work done that bothers them.
>>
>> Although I don't show it, I tense up when the residents approach me when they are covered with food or excrement. Maybe this is what the attendants feel and why they often treat the residents as lepers.
>
> In the following excerpt from the job training study conducted by one of the authors, the observer reflects upon one of his first encounters with a trainee after having spent the initial stages of the research with staff members:
>
>> I approached the two trainees who were working on assembling the radio. The male trainee looked up. I said 'Hi.' He said, 'Hi' and went back to doing what he had been doing. I said, 'Have you built that (the radio) right from scratch?' (After I said this I thought that that was a dumb thing to say or perhaps a very revealing thing to say. Thinking back over the phrase, it came across as perhaps condescending. Asking if he had built it right from scratch might imply that I thought he didn't have the ability. He didn't react in that way but maybe that's the way people think of the 'hard core' unemployed out at the center. Doing well is treated with surprise rather than as standard procedure. Perhaps rather than expecting that they are going to produce and treating

them as if they are going to produce, you treat doing well as a special event.)

The observer thus gained a possible insight into staff members' definitions of trainees through a reflection on his own remark.

(Bogdan and Taylor, 1975, p.67)

It is unusual for field notes to be presented extensively in their original form in research reports. Normally, only brief extracts are given, frequently edited and tidied up. However, it is worth remembering that the field notes are the raw materials from which the evidence provided in many qualitative research reports comes. In assessing those reports we need to be aware of the contingencies of field-note writing (the selectivity involved, the fact that often there is considerable reliance on memory in filling out jotted notes, etc.), and of the filtering process that has taken place between the original field notes and the data presented as evidence in research reports.

Even in the case of documents, data preparation may be necessary before analysis can begin. For example, where they are written in a different language to that in which the analysis is to be carried out and the report written, translation may be required. It may also be necessary to collect contextual information and to add this to documentary material, indicating, for instance, who produced the material and in what circumstances, what any obscure references in the text mean, and so on.

4.2 STARTING THE ANALYSIS

The most obvious difference between analysing unstructured and structured data is that, whereas the latter come ready coded, the former do not. In other words, structured data are collected in a form whose relevance to the focus of the inquiry is obvious (at least if the data collection procedures have been designed properly), so much so that what can and should be done with the data is, to a large extent, a matter of following rules about what sorts of analysis are appropriate given the nature of the data and the purposes of the research. This is not the case with unstructured data, and this is no minor practical consideration for the researcher. The most common question asked by researchers carrying out qualitative data analysis for the first time, and the one that is most difficult to answer, is: now I've got the data, what do I do with them? The reason it is difficult to answer this question is that there is no set of rules, no simple recipe, that one can follow which will always be appropriate and guarantee good results. The task is not just the assignment of data to categories; the categories themselves have to be developed at the same time. In fact, what is involved is a process of mutual fitting between data and categories. There is, then, an essential element of creativity involved, and this is one reason why different researchers working with the same data may produce rather different analyses. Having said this, there are certain general steps that are typically followed in grounded theorizing and the forms of qualitative data analysis analogous to it.

An essential first step is a close reading of the data. This involves looking carefully at the data with a view to identifying aspects of them that may be significant. It is worth emphasizing that, as Henwood and Pidgeon make clear in their Reader article, grounded theorizing is usually associated with research that is exploratory or discovery oriented — for example, ethnographic, participant observation, and life history work. Here the process of analysis is not confined to some particular stage of the research, it begins as soon as the data start to be collected and continues in more or less formal ways through to the completion of the research report. Thus, Howard Becker, a well-known exponent of qualitative method, comments that in participant observation research 'analysis is carried on sequentially, important parts of the analysis being made while the researcher is still gathering his data', and he notes that one of the consequences of this is that 'further data gathering takes its direction from provisional analyses' (Becker, 1970, pp.26–7). This contrasts sharply with research which begins with a set of hypotheses and proceeds to test these. Indeed, such research would normally collect structured data. One of the implications of the exploratory character of qualitative research is that the focus of inquiry is clarified over the course of the data collection and analysis. Furthermore, the analytical categories that are used to make sense of the data (which in the case of hypothesis-testing research are supplied by the hypotheses and the theory lying behind them) have to be developed in the process of data analysis. Indeed, developing such categories is the central task in grounded theorizing.

Usually, the initial close reading of data necessary for this sort of analysis focuses on a sub-sample of the data. This data sample may be chosen haphazardly on the basis of what is most convenient, or those data which look most promising may be selected. Eventually, all the relevant data will be analysed — it is simply a matter of finding a place to start. Reading through the data, the researcher notes down topics or categories to which the data relate and which are relevant to the research focus, or are in some other way interesting or surprising. Annotations are usually made in the margins of the data record, specifying the categories. Also, the researcher is on the look-out for recurrences that may indicate patterns, whether these are typical sequences of events in a setting, or preoccupations around which a particular group's or individual's view of the world revolves.

A next step is often the gathering together of segments of data from different parts of the data record that are relevant to some category. This distinguishes grounded theorizing from some other forms of qualitative data analysis. Some qualitative researchers do not segment and compare data in this way. This is particularly true of those who are concerned with analysing processes of social interaction as in conversation or discourse analysis. For them, segmenting the data and comparing the segments would lose much that is relevant, notably details about the way in which one utterance relates to those before and after it (for instance, the relationship between the interviewer's questions and the informant's answers, how the informant builds on or refers back to things he or she has said earlier, etc.). Here again, the strategies employed depend on the purposes of the research, and the costs and benefits of each strategy must be borne in mind.

The categories produced in the course of coding the data may come from a variety of sources. They may arise from some of the ideas that originally sparked off the research or that set the framework for it, or from more general background knowledge. Perhaps the data seem to confirm the researcher's expectations. But equally, if not more significantly, perhaps they do not. Categories may also arise from the data themselves, in the sense that the people studied may use concepts that seem particularly significant for understanding their behaviour. Good advice that is often given to those engaging in grounded theorizing for the first time is to look out for 'insider' terms — for words and abbreviations that are distinctive to the world that the informant inhabits, and which may appear strange to outsiders. Often these can tell us something about the distinctive ways in which the people we are studying view the world. A classic example is to be found in the study of students in a state medical school in the USA, carried out by Becker and colleagues (Becker et al., 1961). The researchers found that the students used the word 'crock' to describe some patients. For the students a 'crock' was a patient who did not seem to have an identifiable illness and as a result did not constitute a useful case from which the students could learn about the diagnosis and treatment of known illnesses. What the use of that concept suggested was that the students had an instrumental attitude towards patients, viewing them in terms of the opportunities they offered for learning relevant knowledge and skills, rather than primarily as people in need of help. And, indeed, Becker et al. went on to argue that the process of medical education tends to involve a transformation of students' attitudes from the altruism with which they enter medical school towards a more 'professional' orientation.

At the beginning, researchers seek to generate as many categories as possible, not worrying what the relevance of those categories might be to their intended goal. This reflects the creative, exploratory character of the process. Of course, how unconstrained this process of category development should be depends on the purposes of the research and the time constraints under which the researcher is operating. However, generating as many categories as possible is sound advice in many circumstances because it may enable the researcher to see features of the data, or of what the data refer to, that might be overlooked with a more focused approach. Such discoveries can guide the subsequent analysis in two ways. First, they may reveal that there is some doubt about one or more of the assumptions with which the researcher began the analysis. For instance, perhaps the people described are not primarily concerned with what the researcher expected them to be concerned with. Second, it can suggest a quite different focus for the research, one that the researcher judges to be more interesting or significant. (Again, whether or not a researcher can change the research focus, and to what degree, will depend on the constraints under which he or she is working.)

The aim of this sort of initial analysis of unstructured data, then, is to generate categories, each of which collects together several segments of data, some of which look promising as a basis for organizing the analysis and, eventually, the research report. This concern with categories that group many of the data together arises because researchers are usually concerned with stable characteristics or recurrent patterns, not just with what happened at particular points in time; though we noted above that this is not *always* true. The categories may vary in character too, of course. Some may be relatively banal, others may be rather less obvious and more interesting. In Unit 3/4 it was noted that research is judged not only in terms of its validity but also in terms of its relevance, and that one element of this is the extent to which it tells us something new. It follows from this that any novel or theoretically interesting categories that emerge are especially welcome to a researcher. That said, it is rare for such categories to appear immediately or to predominate; and sometimes what appear to be banal categories turn out not to be so at all, while apparently interesting ones prove inapplicable. So, grounded theorizing almost always starts from relatively obvious categories. The goal initially is simply to get a general descriptive sense of the content of the data and how analysis of it might be pursued.

READING

You should now read the short extract by A. Strauss and J. Corbin which is reproduced below. This provides an example of the identification of categories.

LABELING PHENOMENA

We have already remarked on why concepts are the basic units of analysis in the grounded theory method. One can count 'raw' data, but one can't relate or talk about them easily. **Therefore, conceptualizing our data becomes the first step in analysis.** By breaking down and conceptualizing we mean taking apart an observation, a sentence, a paragraph, and giving each discrete incident, idea, or event, a name, something that stands for or represents a phenomenon. Just how do we do this? We ask questions about each one, like: What is this? What does it represent? We compare incident with incident as we go along so that similar phemomena can be given the same name. Otherwise, we would wind up with too many names and very confused!

Let's stop here and take an example. Suppose you are in a fairly expensive but popular restaurant. The restaurant is built on three levels. On the first level is a bar, on the second a small dining area, and on the third, the main dining area and the kitchen. The kitchen is open, so you can see what is going on. Wine, liqueurs, and appropriate glasses in which to serve them are also available on this third level. While waiting for your dinner, you notice a lady in red. She appears to be just standing there in the kitchen, but your common sense tells you that a restaurant wouldn't pay a lady in red just to stand there, especially in a busy kitchen. Your curiosity is piqued, so you decide to do an inductive analysis to see if you can determine just what her job is. (Once a grounded theorist, always a grounded theorist.)

You notice that she is intently looking around the kitchen area, **a work site**, focusing here and then there, taking a mental note of what is going on. *You ask yourself, what is she doing here?* Then you label it **watching**. Watching what? **Kitchen work**.

Next, someone comes up and asks her a question. She answers. This act is different than watching, *so you code it* as **information passing**.

She seems to notice everything. You call this **attentiveness**.

Our lady in red walks up to someone and tells him something. Since this incident also involves information that is passed on, *you also label it*, **information passing**.

Although standing in the midst of all this activity, she doesn't seem to disrupt it. *To describe this phenomenon* you use the term **unintrusiveness**.

She turns and walks quickly and quietly, **efficiency**, into the dining area, and proceeds to **watch**, the activity here also.

She seems to be keeping track of everyone and everything, **monitoring**. But monitoring what? Being an astute observer you notice that she is monitoring the **quality** of the service, how the waiter interacts and responds to the customer; the **timing of service**, how much transpires between seating a customer, their ordering, the delivery of food; and **customer response and satisfaction** with the service.

A waiter comes with an order for a large party, she moves in to help him, **providing assistance**.

The woman looks like she knows what she is doing and is competent at it, **experienced**.

She walks over to a wall near the kitchen and looks at what appears to be a schedule, **information gathering**.

The maitre d' comes down and they talk for a few moments and look around the room for empty tables and judge at what point in the meal the seated customers seem to be: the two are **conferring**.

This example should be sufficient for you to comprehend what we mean by labeling phenomena. It is not unusual for beginning researchers to summarize rather than *conceptualize* data. That is, they merely repeat briefly the gist of the phrase or sentence, but still in a descriptive way. For instance, instead of using a term such as 'conferring' to describe the last incident, they might say something like 'sat and talked to the maitre d'.' Or, use terms such as: 'read the schedule,' 'moved to the dining room,' and 'didn't disrupt.' To invent such phrases doesn't give you a concept to work with. You can see just from this initial coding session that conceptually it is more effective to work with a term such as 'information gathering' rather than 'reading the schedule,' because one might be able to label ten different happenings or events as **information gathering** — her asking a question of one of the chefs, checking on the number of clean glasses, calling a supplier, and so forth.

(Strauss and Corbin, 1990, pp.63–5)

The next step in qualitative data analysis of the kind discussed by Strauss and Corbin is to compare and contrast all the items of data that have been assigned to the same category. Glaser and Strauss refer to this stage as the 'constant comparative method' (Glaser and Strauss, 1967). The aim of this is to clarify what the categories that have emerged mean, as well as to identify sub-categories and relations amongst categories. In the process, these categories may be developed and some data segments may be reassigned as a result. It is then necessary to go through the data sample again in case any data segments not previously identified as relevant have been overlooked. (This is frequently the case.) After this, further data samples will be analysed, perhaps producing new developments in the categories, and these will, of course, make it necessary again to recode previously coded data. What is involved here, then, is an iterative process of analysis which generates categories and interpretations of the data in terms of these categories. And, over time, at least some of the categories will come to be integrated into a network of relationships. These will usually form the core of the main claims of the resulting research report(s).

5 AN EXAMPLE

ACTIVITY 2

(Allow 6 hours for this)

The best way to understand this sort of analysis is to try your hand at it. This is your task here. Enter your word processor, insert your course data disk DATASET, and load the file LYNN.SW2. This is the transcript of the interview contained on Audio-cassette 1. Print out this file. (If for any reason you are unable to use your computer at this point, you will find the transcript in the Audio-Visual Handbook.)

Next, read the brief background information provided in the Audio-Visual Handbook and then listen to the tape, following what is said in the transcript. This will give you a general sense of the content of the interview.

When you have finished doing this, begin reading the transcript again, but this time more slowly. As you do so, stop and make a note of any categories, or what Strauss and Corbin (1990) call 'labels', that occur to you that might help you characterize Lynn's orientation towards her work. The aim is to identify categories that seem to collect together things she says and does in a way that makes sense of how she relates to patients, colleagues, her conditions of work, etc.

Complete this activity before you read on.

In our analysis of this interview we produced quite a large number of categories of various kinds, as you probably did too. Some of them were to do with kinds of patients, and of these many were related to medical conditions (patients who had had cerebro-vascular accidents; patients with diabetes, thyroid problems, or strokes; and geriatric patients, for instance), but others were not medical in any direct sense (patients in the older age group, active patients, intelligent patients, patients with social problems, for instance). We also found another set of categories that seemed to refer to sorts of action on the part of medical staff, including Lynn herself (nursing/physical care, education, intensive care, designating responsibility for a patient to a particular nurse, one-to-one treatment, allocation to a high dependency room or a single room, allocation to a geriatric ward, etc). Another set of categories referred to what we might think of as constraints operating on nurses — for example, number of beds in a ward, etc.

These by no means exhaust the categories that you might have found, but they indicate some of the main possibilities.

ACTIVITY 3

(Spend up to 2 hours on this)

You may have noticed that, in presenting our categories, we have already identified some relationships among them, notably in seeing most of our categories as falling under three main headings (types of patient, types of medical action, types of constraint). You may have done the same, but it is just as likely that, instead, you have generated rather a lot of categories without specifying relationships amongst them. If you are in this position, look back at your categories and see if you can find any relationships that might enable you to structure your categories in a more economical way. Alternatively, look at the categories you have and pick out a small number, say five or six, that seem to you to be important or interesting, or that have the largest number of pieces of data listed under them. For the next part of the analysis you will need to work with this small number of categories.

Using your annotated transcript, identify the first piece of text that you have coded under one of your categories, and then copy and store it on disk in a separate file with the relevant category's name. Go through all of the transcript doing the same for each piece of text that is relevant to one of your categories.

At the end you should have a small number of new files each containing data relevant to one of your categories. When you have reached this point, print out each of your category files.

The next step in the analysis is to look at the data we have filed under the same heading. Let us begin with the data relating to our heading: 'types of patient'. There are many types of patient mentioned, but we shall concentrate on just seven of them: cerebro-vascular accident, diabetic, myocardial infarction, older age group, strokes, thyroid and geriatric. We have printed out the data we coded under each of our headings and have included them in Appendix 1. You might like to look at this briefly before reading on.

The general category 'types of patient' arises very much from the questions that Senga asked Lynn, of course, and it is fairly obvious that this category would be important. What we need to ask when looking at these data, though, is: what is the organizing principle behind Lynn's use of the various sub-categories? Where the categories are medical, we might be tempted to suppose that this principle relates to medical knowledge about different types of illness, so that we might get a form of organization something like that shown in Table 1.

Table 1 Medical diagnoses

Heart problems	Problems of the brain and nervous system	Other
Myocardial infarction	Cerebro-vascular accident	Diabetes
	Stroke	Thyroid

However, we must take care not to jump to conclusions here. We are making the assumption that nurses and doctors operate primarily, if not exclusively, on the basis of medical considerations. Instead of assuming this, we need to look carefully at what Lynn actually says. And doing this, it seems to us that a structure more like that shown in Table 2 emerges.

Table 2 Length of intensive nursing care required

Short	Longer	Very long
Diabetics	Cerebro-vascular accident	Geriatric
Thyroid patients	Stroke victims	Older age groups
Myocardial infarction		

One of Lynn's central concerns seems to be how much intensive nursing or physical care patients need, and she distinguishes among patients in large part on this basis. Much of what she says in the interview can be interpreted as relating to this concern. It seems that she monitors how many patients needing intensive nursing care there are on the ward at any one time, presumably because her nurses simply cannot cope with more than a certain number. She indicates what she means by needing intensive care: these are patients who are not 'up and about', they are not 'mobile', they need feeding, they need close observation and so forth. This concern also underlies her use of the category 'geriatric'. The problem with the patients falling under this category, from her point of view, is that they require a high level of physical care *and* they are likely to need this for a long time. Furthermore, interestingly, we find that this category, though apparently medical, is not purely medical in meaning. Whether someone is classified as geriatric, and whether the geriatric consultant is brought in with a view to arranging transfer to a geriatric ward, depends on social as well as medical factors; in particular, on whether there is someone at home who can look after the patient.

What we have here is a theme that could form a central organizing principle of a research report based on analysis of these data; though, of course, much further work would need to be done on it. However, it is clearly not the only possible organizing theme — not all of our categories relate to it in any very obvious way. It seems to be an important starting point, though.

Let us look at one more of the categories we developed, one of a rather different kind. There were a number of places in the interview where it seemed to us that Lynn was concerned about the implications of what she was describing, either for her own image as a caring professional or for the reputation of the hospital. We have listed the items of data that we classified under the heading of 'Concern with image' in Appendix 2. (You might like to look at this briefly now before reading on.)

In these extracts, Lynn seems to be anticipating how Senga, and probably others listening to the audio-tape as well, may evaluate her comments. She is perhaps aware that it may appear as though decisions are being made by her that are based not so much on patient need as on what is most convenient for herself, her staff and the hospital. She seems to try to counter this by various means. For example, she indicates that it is not *her* decision but someone else's, as in the use of 70 as the cut-off age for allocation to the coronary unit and the decision to send patients to geriatric wards. At the same time, she attempts to reassure us that these decisions are not harmful to patients' needs, the age cut-off 'works quite well' and 'has not caused any great problems'. Similarly, she points out that the geriatric wards have better resources for rehabilitation than do medical wards. This 'concern with image' category is more like the sort that a discourse analyst would be interested in — it relates to the talk itself rather than involving inference from what is said in the interview to what people actually say and do in the world, in this case on the ward. At the same time, it has obvious links with our earlier theme.

ACTIVITY 4

(Allow up to 6 hours for this)

Carefully examine the data you have listed under each of the categories you selected in the previous activity. Consider how you would define these categories, whether there are sub-categories within them, whether they seem to be related to other categories, and so on. Take some time over this.

When you have finished, listen to the remainder of the audio-cassette, on which Senga Bond reflects on her research and provides a preliminary analysis of the interview data and of some observational data that she collected.

On the basis of this example of qualitative data analysis, we can identify a number of features to add to our earlier discussion. First, it is worth thinking a little more about the character of the categories we have developed. One thing to notice is that, in our analysis, we did not assign all the data to our categories; in other words, the categorization was not exhaustive. For some purposes, categorization systems may need to be exhaustive, but usually they do not have to be. Also important is that the categories we developed are not mutually exclusive; in other words, sometimes the same segment of data is listed under more than one heading. Again, for some purposes it may be necessary to develop categories that are mutually exclusive, but for the sort of analysis characteristic of grounded theorizing it is not. It should also be noted that our allocation of data to categories is not very rigorous: the categories are not clearly defined with specific criteria indicating the sort of data which should and should not be included. The goal of grounded theorizing is to facilitate more rigorous definition of categories *through* the process of analysis, rather than specifying what categories are appropriate and how these are to be defined at the *beginning* of the research process, as in hypothesis-testing research.

Certainly, in the initial stages of qualitative data analysis, the concern is with collecting some items of data together that seem to belong with one another in certain respects, with a view to understanding what their similarities are. For this reason, you may not agree that all of the items we listed under a particular heading belong there, and you may have put some others under that heading that we did not, as well as developing some headings that were different to ours. There is also a question about how much of the surrounding context one should include in the data extracts. For example, in the case of interview data, should one always include the questions asked, to which what the informant says is a response? These are matters of judgement. On the one hand, some context will be necessary to make the extract intelligible (while one can always look back to the original data to understand the context, doing this every time would be too time consuming). On the other hand, the longer each data extract is the more cumbersome the analysis becomes. Some happy medium is desirable.

Another point is that, even working with the relatively small amount of data contained in the interview, you will probably have become aware of one of the practical problems involved in grounded theorizing. Using a word processor to copy, file and print out segments of data relevant to particular categories is certainly a lot easier than copying segments of data by hand or cutting and sticking segments on to cards — methods that were used in the past. However, it is still time consuming. As a result, a number of computer programs have been specially developed for carrying out this sort of analysis (see Tesch, 1990; Fielding and Lee, 1991; Dey, 1992).

Earlier, we noted that analysis of unstructured data could be directed towards a variety of types of intended product. A related dimension concerns how far the sort of analysis we have outlined above is pursued. The analysis we have carried out here is quite limited in character, and it would be difficult to go much beyond this solely on the basis of the data we have. Of course, usually researchers have a much larger amount of data and this may allow much greater development of our understanding of the perspectives and behaviour of the people concerned. Equally, if we also have observational data we may be able to look at the relationship between what the informants say they do and what they actually seem to do, etc. (as Senga Bond was able to do). Strauss and Corbin (1990) provide a clear account of one direction that this further analysis can take, involving the development of a dense and well-integrated theory. Another is towards providing the basis for a quantitative analysis, but this requires the development of the categories into mutually exclusive types that can form the basis for counting instances or even for developing scales. Which of these directions is most appropriate depends on the purposes of the research and the nature of the data.

Our discussion has been concerned with qualitative data analysis dealing with a single case and devoted to describing or explaining some of the features of that case. Qualitative data analysis is usually associated with a case study approach, as described in Unit 7. However, this often involves collecting data on several cases. Sometimes data on these cases will be pooled and the sort of analysis we have discussed here will be applied to the whole corpus. At other times, separate analyses will be carried out on each case, the aim perhaps being to develop and test theoretical ideas further through systematic comparison of strategically selected cases. Equally, sometimes the categories developed in one case will be applied to another simply to illuminate similarities and differences. A variety of approaches has been used.

6 REFLEXIVITY AND THE ASSESSMENT OF VALIDITY

The process of data analysis produces the main claims that form the core of research reports. And in qualitative research the evidence that is presented by the researcher in support of claims will be a selection from the segments of data collected together as relevant to the categories that form part of those claims. However, of course, claims are not assessed only in terms of the evidence offered in support of them but also in terms of credibility, against the background of information about how the research was carried out and the likelihood of error that this implies. Such considerations should also be taken into account by the researcher engaging in qualitative data analysis. In deciding what are and are not reasonable inferences to be made on the basis of her or his data, the researcher must consider the likelihood of errors of various kinds. For instance, does it seem likely that the data may have been shaped by the presence of the researcher in such a fashion as to lead to misleading conclusions? This is the problem of reactivity again. Were the people observed 'putting on a show' or 'maintaining a front' for the observer? Did the informant simply tell the researcher what he or she thought the researcher wanted to hear? Similarly, how complex and uncertain in validity are the judgements likely to have been that produced the data? Was the observer or informant in a position to be able to observe and record accurately what happened? Were the phenomena being described of a kind that anyone would probably be able to recognize and agree on, or were they more problematic? Equally, is there any indication that the observer or the informant could have been biased, consciously or unconsciously selecting evidence to support one outcome rather than another? As readers, we need to look for the extent to which the researcher seems to have been aware of potential sources of error, and what he or she did to counter these, as well as considering them for ourselves.

Consideration of the process of research and its possible implications for the validity of the main claims and conclusions of a study is one part of what is sometimes referred to as reflexivity (Hammersley and Atkinson, 1983). What is proposed is that the researcher should be a reflective practitioner, continually thinking about the process of research and especially about her or his own role in it, and the implications of this for the analysis. As we noted earlier, qualitative researchers usually record in their field notes their interpretations of and feelings about what they observe and about their role. And this process of reflection is often continued throughout the whole process of the research.

An equally important aspect of reflexivity is that the process by which the data and findings were produced should be made sufficiently explicit for a reader to make a reasonable assessment of the credibility of the findings. Of course, the information about the research that we have available to us as readers will always be quite limited. It will also vary a great deal between research reports. Not surprisingly, book-length reports tend to provide more information than do articles. However, sometimes we are able to track down other reports arising from the same piece of research and these may give us extra information. Furthermore, as we mentioned in Section 3, occasionally a reflexive account or natural history of the research will be available and this may provide very useful background information on the basis of which to assess the claims made by the researcher.

In Unit 3/4 it was noted that researchers may sometimes provide reports of attempts at respondent validation and triangulation. These are useful further sources of information, especially where the claims made are very controversial. Indeed, evidence of this kind may occasionally be crucial for the assessment of the findings of qualitative research. However, as was made clear in that earlier unit, such evidence, like that of other kinds, is never absolutely conclusive. It must be interpreted and assessed, and there is usually scope for conflicting judgements about it.

7 CONCLUSION

In this unit we have looked at some of the strategies used by qualitative researchers for analysing unstructured data. We concentrated in particular on the kind of qualitative data analysis that has been codified by Glaser and Strauss (1967) as grounded theorizing, since this represents probably the most common approach in use today. We have only been able to provide an outline here of what is involved in this sort of analysis. However, it should provide you with a clear sense of the sort of analytical work that underlies qualitative research reports, and facilitate your assessments of the claims they make.

FURTHER READING

Many introductions to qualitative or ethnographic social research include some discussion of qualitative data analysis. See, for example:

Hammersley, M. and Atkinson, P. (1983) *Ethnography: Principles in Practice*, London, Tavistock.

Lofland, J. and Lofland, L. (1984) *Analyzing Social Settings*, Belmont, CA, Wadsworth.

There are also some books devoted entirely to this subject. See, for instance:

Strauss, A. and Corbin, J. (1990) *Basics of Qualitative Research: Grounded Theory Procedures and Techniques*, Newbury Park, CA, Sage:

> This is the best of the books on grounded theorizing as regards how to do it. The initial chapters provide a very straightforward introduction.

Strauss, A. (1987) *Qualitative Analysis for Social Scientists*, New York, Cambridge University Press:

> This book represents the same approach as that of Strauss and Corbin above, but is somewhat more advanced and difficult to follow.

Glaser, B.G. and Strauss, A.L. (1967) *The Discovery of Grounded Theory*, Chicago, IL, Aldine:

> This is the original book on grounded theorizing. It has since been superseded by the above except that it indicates something of the original motivation for this approach.

On the use of microcomputers in handling qualitative data, see:

Tesch, R. (1990) *Qualitative Research: Analysis Types and Software Tools*, Lewes, Falmer Press.

Fielding, N.G. and Lee, R.M. (eds) (1991) *Using Computers in Qualitative Research*, London, Sage.

The following serves simultaneously as an introduction to qualitative data analysis and to the use of microcomputers in this:

Dey, I. (1992) *Qualitative Data Analysis*, London, Routledge.

REFERENCES

Becker, H.S. (1970) *Sociological Work*, London, Allen Lane.

Becker, H.S., Geer, B., Hughes, E.C. and Strauss, A.L. (1961) *Boys in White: Student Culture in Medical School*, Chicago, IL, University of Chicago Press.

Billig, M. (1991) *Ideology and Opinions: Studies in Rhetorical Psychology*, London, Sage.

Boelen, W.A.M. (1992) '*Street Corner Society*: Cornerville revisited', *Journal of Contemporary Ethnography*, vol. 21, no. 1, pp.11–51.

Bogdan, R.C. and Taylor, S. (1975) *Introduction to Qualitative Research Methods*, New York, Wiley.

Bryman, A. (1988) *Quality and Quantity in Social Research*, London, Allen and Unwin.

Cornwell, J. (1990) *A Thief in the Night: The Death of Pope John Paul I*, Harmondsworth, Penguin.

Delamont, S. and Hamilton, D. (1984) 'Revisiting classroom research: a continuing cautionary tale', in Delamont, S. (ed.) *Readings on Interaction in the Classroom*, London, Methuen.

Dey, I. (1992) *Qualitative Data Analysis*, London, Routledge.

Fielding, N.G. and Lee, R.M. (eds) (1991) *Using Computers in Qualitative Research*, London, Sage.

Frake, C.O. (1980) *Language and Cultural Description*, Stanford, CA, Stanford University Press (extract reproduced in Offprints Booklet 4).

French, J. and French, P. (1984) 'Gender imbalances in the primary classroom: an interactional account', *Educational Research*, vol. 26, no. 2 (reproduced in Offprints Booklet 1).

Glaser, B.G. and Strauss, A.L. (1967) *The Discovery of Grounded Theory*, Chicago, IL, Aldine.

Goodwin, C. (1981) *Conversational Organisation*, New York, Academic Press.

Hammersley, M. (1980) *A Peculiar World? Teaching and Learning in an Inner City School*, unpublished PhD thesis, University of Manchester.

Hammersley, M. (1992) *What's Wrong with Ethnography?*, London, Routledge.

Hammersley, M. (ed.) (1993) *Social Research: Philosophy, Politics and Practice*, London, Sage (DEH313 Reader).

Hammersley, M. and Atkinson, P. (1983) *Ethnography: Principles in Practice*, London, Tavistock.

Henwood, K.L. and Pidgeon, N.F. (1992) 'Qualitative research and psychological theorizing', in Hammersley, M. (ed.) (1993) (DEH313 Reader).

Krieger, S. (1979) 'Research and the construction of a text', in Denzin, N.K. (ed.) *Studies in Symbolic Interaction*, vol. 2, Greenwich, CT, JAI Press.

McIntyre, D. and Macleod, G. (1978) 'The characteristics and uses of systematic classroom observation', in McAleese, R. and Hamilton, D. (eds) *Understanding Classroom Life*, Slough, NFER.

Ochs, E. (1979) 'Transcription as theory', in Ochs, E. and Schiefflin, B. (eds) *Developmental Pragmatics*, New York, Academic Press.

Potter, J. and Wetherell, M. (1987) *Discourse and Social Psychology*, London, Sage.

Punch, M. (1979) *Policing the Inner City*, London and Basingstoke, Macmillan (extract reproduced in Offprints Booklet 4).

Schegloff, E.A. (1971) 'Notes on a conversational practice: formulating place', in Sudnow, D. (ed.) *Studies in Social Interaction*, New York, Free Press.

Smith, J.K. and Heshusius, L. (1986) 'Closing down the conversation: the end of the quantitative–qualitative debate among educational inquirers', *Educational Researcher*, vol. 15, no. 1, pp.4–12.

Strauss, A. and Corbin, J. (1990) *Basics of Qualitative Research: Grounded Theory Procedures and Techniques*, Newbury Park, CA, Sage.

Tesch, R. (1990) *Qualitative Research: Analysis Types and Software Tools*, Lewes, Falmer Press.

Walford, G. (ed.) (1987) *Doing Sociology of Education*, Lewes, Falmer.

Walker, J.C. and Evers, C.W. (1988) 'The epistemological unity of educational research', in Keeves, J.P. (ed.) *Educational Research, Methodology and Measurement: An International Handbook*, Oxford, Pergamon.

Whyte, W.F. (1981) *Street Corner Society*, 3rd edn, Chicago, IL, University of Chicago Press.

Whyte, W.F. (1992) 'In defence of *Street Corner Society*', *Journal of Contemporary Ethnography*, vol. 21, no. 1, pp.52–68.

Wuebben, P.L., Straits, B.C. and Schulman, G.I. (1974) *The Experiment as a Social Occasion*, Berkeley, CA, Glendessary Press.

ACKNOWLEDGEMENTS

Grateful acknowledgement is made to the following sources for permission to reproduce material in this unit:

Hammersley, M. and Atkinson, P. (1983) *Ethnography: Principles In Practice*, Tavistock Publications, © Martyn Hammersley and Paul Atkinson; Strauss, A. and Corbin, J. (1990) *Basics of Qualitative Research*, Sage Publications Inc.

APPENDIX 1

(From the transcripts of the interviews recorded on Audio-cassette 1. Presenter: Senga Bond, interviewee: Lynn Sadler.)

CEREBRO-VASCULAR ACCIDENT

S.B.: One, one point you made here was that your work varies a lot depending on the kinds of patients that you have. Can you tell me a little bit how, how this happens?

L.S.: Yes, em, it's particularly increased if you have patients who've had cerebro-vascular accidents, em initially when they come in they're generally very ill.

S.B.: Mm.

L.S.: Em, they may be to the point of course of being unconscious and needing intensive care really, em, unfortunately we don't have the staff to do it on a one-to-one basis, but obviously you've got to, to give a specific nurse that patient to look after for her span of duty. Em, but also they become as you get them over that stage, rehabilitation plays a very, very much a part in recovery. Compared to somebody like, em, a diabetic who once you've got over the ill stage perhaps if they've come in in a coma, they're up and about the ward, em, don't need nursing on a one-to-one basis, apart from education.

S.B.: Uhuh.

L.S.: Em, and that really is not care in the physical sense, it's more talking to them and describing things.

S.B.: Uhuh.

L.S.: Em, so it depends, you see if you've maybe got six patients in who have got cerebro-vascular accidents, that immediately they need more care, not more care but, well, yes more care than perhaps your diabetics or your thyroid patients who are up and about the ward who perhaps from a nursing point of view you're not doing that much for during the day sort of thing, you know. But that's how it comes to vary.

S.B.: Mm, you mentioned, em, patients being poorly. Em, describe a patient when they're poorly. Can you do that?

L.S.: Em, yes ... It's going to vary really with different conditions, but em, I class it really by somebody who's going to need closer observation than the rest of the patients. Em, and that's the sort of patient that I would put into a high dependency room. It may be somebody who is unconscious, em, if they've had a cerebro-vascular accident, we do get overdoses and that in as well, it may be somebody who's in a diabetic coma.

DIABETIC

L.S.: Compared to somebody like, em, a diabetic who once you've got over the ill stage perhaps if they've come in in a coma, they're up and about the ward, em, don't need nursing on a one-to-one basis, apart from education.

S.B.:	Uhuh.
L.S.:	Em, and that really is not care in the physical sense, it's more talking to them and describing things.
S.B.:	Uhuh.
	Em, so it depends, you see if you've maybe got six patients in who have got cerebro-vascular accidents, that immediately they need more care, not more care but, well, yes more care than perhaps your diabetics or your thyroid patients who are up and about the ward who perhaps from a nursing point of view you're not doing that much for during the day sort of thing, you know. But that's how it comes to vary.
S.B.:	Mm, you mentioned, em, patients being poorly. Em, describe a patient when they're poorly. Can you do that?
L.S.:	Em, yes ... It's going to vary really with different conditions, but, em, I class it really by somebody who's going to need closer observation than the rest of the patients. Em, and that's the sort of patient that I would put into a high dependency room. It may be somebody who is unconscious, em, if they've had a cerebro-vascular accident, we do get overdoses and that in as well, it may be somebody who's in a diabetic coma.
S.B.:	Uhuh.
L.S.:	So there's some real significant problem that maybe just as an experienced nurse you tell without actually having done anything by looking at them. They may be having breathing problems, em, their colour maybe, you know, shocking. Em, they may be sweaty, em, they just look, they look ill. Em, when you come to do observations they may have a very high or very low blood pressure, mental state as well also needs assessing and they may be very confused and in fact to be put in another room is maybe going to make them worse and upset other patients you've got to sort of put them in a single room where you can watch them closely. Em, they may be in a lot of pain depending on their condition, they may have a paralysis, em, they may need, em, intravenous therapy and this sort of thing. That's not always a guideline to how ill they are, em, but you know they may need airways in or they may need suction if they're unconscious. That's the sort of patient that I class as poorly.
L.S.:	Em, they may be to the point of course of being unconscious and needing intensive care really, em, unfortunately we don't have the staff to do it on a one-to-one basis, but obviously you've got to, to give a specific nurse that patient to look after for her span of duty. Em, but also they become, as you get them over that stage, rehabilitation plays a very, very much a part in recovery. Compared to somebody like, em, a diabetic who once you've got over the ill stage perhaps if they've come in in a coma, they're up and about the ward, em, don't need nursing on a one-to-one basis, apart from education.
S.B.:	Uhuh.
L.S.:	Em, and that really is not care in the physical sense, it's more talking to them and describing things.
L.S.:	Em, ... you, we tend to get an older age group as well of course, medical wards do, pneumonias and this type of thing tend to affect an older age population and you can sometimes get a lot of social

problems and this type of thing that, em, need more involvement from a nursing aspect. You've got to have more input into these type of patients. Em, so it depends, you see if you've maybe got six patients in who have got cerebro-vascular accidents, that immediately they need more care, not more care but, well, yes more care than perhaps your diabetics or your thyroid patients who are up and about the ward who perhaps from a nursing point of view you're not doing that much for during the day sort of thing, you know. But that's how it comes to vary.

MYOCARDIAL INFARCTION

L.S.: Really once you've got strokes over this, em, phase and they're up and about, em, you know, they change, you can tell again. Em, what else do we have really, em ... Quite a lot of things, you know we have quite a quick turnover, myocardial infarctions and that, once you've got them over the poorly episode if they're ill when they come in, usually within a couple of days they're up and about as well.

S.B.: Do you have them directly, or do they come from a coronary care unit?

L.S.: Em, we have an age-cut off for myocardial infarctions. Well anybody with a heart condition. Em, anybody under 70 goes to the coronary care unit where they spend 48 hours and then they come back to you.

S.B.: Mm.

L.S.: Anybody over 70 comes directly to the ward.

S.B.: And why is that?

L.S.: Purely because the coronary care unit only has six beds and they cannot cater for every patient who's had a myocardial infarction and it's just unfortunate that they think that the younger people should have the closer observation from direct monitoring. Em, that doesn't always follow, if we've had a patient who's been 70 plus who perhaps develops arythmia.

S.B.: Yes.

L.S.: Em, and they do have a bed in the coronary care unit then they will admit that patient, but the unfortunate thing is, if they then get somebody of 28, 30 who's had a myocardial infarction then the older patients are moved out to accommodate the under 70s. It works quite well but, you know, I don't think it's ever been a great problem of the age cut-off, but the reason is they just couldn't cope with every patient.

OLDER AGE GROUP

L.S.: Em, ... you, we tend to get an older age group as well of course, medical wards do, pneumonias and this type of thing tend to affect an older age population and you can sometimes get a lot of social problems and this type of thing that, em, need more involvement from a nursing aspect. You've got to have more input into these type of patients. Em, so it depends, you see if you'maybe got six patients in who have got cerebro-vascular accidents, that immediately they need more care, not more care but, well, yes more care than perhaps your diabetics or your thyroid patients who are up and about the ward who perhaps from a nursing point of view you're not doing that much for during the day sort of thing, you know. But that's how it comes to vary.

L.S.: Em, and they do have a bed in the coronary care unit then they will admit that patient, but the unfortunate thing is, if they then get somebody of 28, 30 who's had a myocardial infarction then the older patients are moved out to accommodate the under 70s. It works quite well but, you know, I don't think it's ever been a great problem of the age cut-off, but the reason is they just couldn'cope with every patient.

L.S.: Unfortunately it was full and the waiting list for this was a very long time so we actually rehabilitated her as much as we possibly could on the ward and in fact she's been discharged home now. Em, but we tend to just have isolated cases like that. Em, we did have a gentleman who was about the same age who we had in for about four months as well, but usually if they are older than that they go to one of the long-stay wards. So it's a fairly rare occurrence for that to happen. You know, we still have them up to about three months, but half a year is a long time on my particular ward.

STROKES

L.S.: Really. Once you've got strokes over this, em, phase and they're up and about, em, you know, they change, you can tell again. Em, what else do we have really, em.

S.B.: Do you, do you find you have different likes and dislikes in relation to the kind of intensity of nursing that you have to give?

L.S.: Eh, no, not really. I like it varied. No, there's nothing specific. The only thing that I find is a problem morale-wise, is if you get somebody in who is perhaps not progressing as well as you would like them to. An ideal example of that is somebody who's had a stroke.

S.B.: Yes.

L.S.: And, em, they're not getting over their paralysis and the patient is getting very low, em, you know, 'Oh I'm not getting any better' type of thing. Em, and it transmits to the nurses as well.

S.B.: Mm.

L.S.: Because the nurses say, well, why isn't he getting better and it's trying to keep morale up and this type of thing. I think that can be a disappointing aspect at some time.

S.B.: So is this not unusual to have patients in for four or five months?

L.S.: Em, it's fairly unusual for that length of time, yes, em, the reason why it happened in this particular case was the lady was 60 and she previously, she had a very severe stroke, it actually affected both sides of her body and, em, she was a very very active lady, em, prior to admission and she really was in no way a geriatric patient although we knew for a fact she was going to be a long-stay patient and to have gone to a long-stay ward really wouldn't have done her any good at all, in fact I think it might have been detrimental.

S.B.: Yes.

L.S.: Now the only other ward was this young chronic sick ward.

S.B.: Uhuh.

L.S.: Unfortunately it was full and the waiting list for this was a very long time so we actually rehabilitated her as much as we possibly could on the ward and in fact she's been discharged home now. Em, but we tend to just have isolated cases like that. Em, we did have a gentleman who was about the same age who we had in for about four months as well, but usually if they are older than that they go to one of the long-stay wards. So it's a fairly rare occurrence for that to happen. You know, we still have them up to about three months, but half a year is a long time on my particular ward.

L.S.: In that way they are getting some supervision from the hospital so that if things start to break down at home we know about them directly. Em, other things, em, we may get somebody in who is a stroke who is progressing very well but needs more rehabilitation so that the consultant might feel in fact that they are going to benefit from hospital admission for a couple of weeks, particularly with a view to daily living assessment because they have kitchens and things over there where they can actually be seen to how they're going to cope in household activities before being discharged, so they may in fact, they may go over there for a period of assessment for a week before being discharged.

S.B.: I thought then we could start off by discussing the patient that you had, that we discussed in the first interview who was a patient you'd had in for about five months who had a severe stroke.

L.S.: Yes.

S.B.: And you kept her for that length of time.

L.S.: Yes.

S.B.: And you said at that time that she was in no way a geriatric patient.

L.S.: Yes.

S.B.: You didn't want to send her to a geriatric ward, you kept her for a long time on this ward. What made you think that she wasn't a geriatric patient? What was it about her?

L.S.: Em, it may have been her age to a certain extent because I, personally I tend to think of sort of 70, the late sixties, seventies as classing into the old age problems, em, this lady was 61 and, I mean I know you can get a lot of 80-year-olds that are very alert but mentally she was, and knowing some of the geriatric wards that I've actually seen we felt that this particular lady may have run into problems had she been in with patients that were perhaps in a worse condition than she was. Em, patients with communication problems and things. She needed people, we felt, about her own age, or younger, who in fact could stimulate her and in fact help her. She was a very intelligent lady, em, she'd been a semi-professional flower arranger, em, and it was a combined discussion it wasn't just between nurses and doctors but it was with physiotherapists and the occupational therapist. And in fact the geriatric consultant himself felt that one of his long-stay wards would not be the answer for this particular patient. We were talking about, em, long-term hospitalization and you find that, em, the sort of patients which are on, who are on long-term geriatric wards are, em, perhaps patients who've had strokes, who have very severe strokes, a lot of them of course are very elderly, em, maybe senile dementia patients, em, incontinent patients, and we felt that these sort of surroundings were, were not going to help this patient at all.

L.S.: That's right. They also have a day hospital, a geriatric day hospital, so if for instance we have somebody, we cover quite a wide variety you see. It may be sort of things such as a cerebral tumours, it could be strokes, it could be cardiac problems, respiratory problems. Em, if we feel in fact that they could cope at home, they may be living with daughters, sons but that they do need some relief or do need some hospital supervision but it doesn't need to be full term, we discharge them home and perhaps they come back to the day hospital two or three times a week, once a week.

L.S.: Em, well social conditions are one if, em, we are running into problems because a patient is not able to cope at all, em, at home and is in unsuitable conditions, you know, perhaps, em, self neglect and this sort of thing, has no family or has a family who are not able to give us any assistance, that is one reason for a referral. It may be because of medical problems, em, depending on their condition, if they're going to need long-term care, a stroke for example.

THYROID

L.S.: Em, so it depends, you see if you've maybe got six patients in who have got cerebro-vascular accidents, that immediately they need more care, not more care but, well, yes more care than perhaps your diabetics or your thyroid patients who are up and about the ward who perhaps from a nursing point of view you're not doing that much for during the day sort of thing, you know. But that's how it comes to vary.

GERIATRIC

L.S.: Em, it's fairly unusual for that length of time, yes, em, the reason why it happened in this particular case was the lady was 60 and she previously, she had a very severe stroke, it actually affected both sides of her body and, em, she was a very very active lady, em, prior to admission and she really was in no way a geriatric patient although we knew for a fact she was going to be a long-stay patient and to have gone to a long-stay ward really wouldn't have done her any good at all, in fact I think it might have been detrimental.

S.B.: This lady who was the long-term patient who very nicely went home. You said she was in no way a geriatric patient. How would you describe a patient who would fall into that category?

L.S.: I think it's very difficult because there is no laid down, em, rules. What they tend to do actually is go by age which doesn't always fit in, em, because they tend to use 65 as the age of classing onwards as geriatric patients, but you can get some 70-year-olds who are very, very sharp and alert, em, but within my own particular ward we tend to refer patients who are over 65 years of age who are going to need longer treatment. Em, maybe for rehabilitation because the actual, em, geriatric wards they have short-stay wards which are for rehabilitation or longer-stay wards.

S.B.: Mm mm.

L.S.: Now if we've got somebody who's maybe 70 and who just needs rehabilitation with a view to going home but perhaps needs to be in hospital a few more weeks, em, we'll refer them to the consultant who is in charge of that area. And likewise, if we have somebody who is from poor social circumstances who is not going to be able to cope on their own who really doesn't warrant a hospital admission

	long term then again the consultant actually from that area comes and assesses them for the ward. So in fact they assess the patient rather than us, the consultant comes across and sees them whilst they're still on my ward and allocates the ward that he would like them to go to and it's worked on that basis.
S.B.:	So it's the geriatric consultant ... (L.S.: that's right, yes). What, what kind of things would suggest that you would refer a patient for this consultation, because obviously it's a two way (L.S.: yes) thing. You suggest they come and see them. (L.S.: Yes.) With a view perhaps to making a decision.
L.S.:	That's right. They also have a day hospital, a geriatric day hospital, so if for instance we have somebody, we cover quite a wide variety you see. It may be sort of things such as a cerebral tumours, it could be strokes, it could be cardiac problems, respiratory problems. Em, if we feel in fact that they could cope at home, they may be living with daughters, sons but that they do need some relief or do need some hospital supervision but it doesn't need to be full term, we discharge them home and perhaps they come back to the day hospital two or three times a week, once a week.
S.B.:	Yes.
L.S.:	In that way they are getting some supervision from the hospital so that if things start to break down at home we know about them directly. Em, other things, em, we may get somebody in who is a stroke who is progressing very well but needs more rehabilitation so that the consultant might feel in fact that they are going to benefit from hospital admission for a couple of weeks, particularly with a view to daily living assessment because they have kitchens and things over there where they can actually be seen to how they're going to cope in household activities before being discharged, so they may in fact, they may go over there for a period of assessment for a week before being discharged.
S.B.:	Yes, yes.
L.S.:	But as I said if you get somebody with poor social circumstances or who is going not going to cope at all then they're the patients who would go on for longer care.
S.B.:	I thought then we could start off by discussing the patient that you had, that we discussed in the first interview who was a patient you'd had in for about five months who had a severe stroke.
L.S.:	Yes.
S.B.:	And you kept her for that length of time.
L.S.:	Yes.
S.B.:	And you said at that time that she was in no way a geriatric patient.
L.S.:	Yes.
S.B.:	You didn't want to send her to a geriatric ward, you kept her for a long time on this ward. What made you think that she wasn't a geriatric patient? What was it about her?
L.S.:	Em, it may have been her age to a certain extent because I, personally I tend to think of sort of 70, the late 60s, 70s as classing into the old age problems, em, this lady was 61 and, I mean I know you can get a lot of 80-year-olds that are very alert but mentally she was, and knowing some of the geriatric wards that I've actually seen we felt that this particular lady may have run into problems had she been in with patients that were perhaps in a worse condition than she was. Em, patients with communication problems and things. She needed

people, we felt, about her own age, or younger, who in fact could stimulate her and in fact help her. She was a very intelligent lady, em, she'd been a semi-professional flower arranger, em, and it was a combined discussion it wasn't just between nurses and doctors but it was with physiotherapists and the occupational therapist. And in fact the geriatric consultant himself felt that one of his long-stay wards would not be the answer for this particular patient. We were talking about, em, long-term hospitalization and you find that, em, the sort of patients which are on, who are on long-term geriatric wards are, em, perhaps patients who've had strokes, who have very severe strokes, a lot of them of course are very elderly, em, maybe senile dementia patients, em, incontinent patients, and we felt that these sort of surroundings were, were not going to help this patient at all.

S.B.: Have you any patients in just now that you would describe as being geriatric?

L.S.: Yes, we've got a couple, em. We've got one lady who's been with us for about two weeks I think now, she's a lady in her 80s who, em, does have senile dementia. She's been diagnosed as having that but it's not very obvious while she's in the ward but her husband does say that she's not capable of, em, organizing any home care or cooking or anything like that when she's at home, and she never knows what day of the week or whatever it is. Em, she's a lady who's not mobile, she needs total nursing care, we need to feed her as well. Em, her husband has got great problems with her at home. He's got to the stage now where he can't cope with her because he himself has had an amputation of one of his legs this year. Em, and he says he manages just to look after himself and the house and keep his wife reasonably clean, but that's about all, and it's been getting extremely difficult for him a few weeks prior to admission. She's been having a series of falls and in fact it was this last fall that brought her into hospital. So I think all things told he and his wife were running into great difficulties at home. She may benefit from some, which we are trying to at the moment, some rehabilitation maybe over a period of weeks where we can maybe get her mobile again. But I think we're going to be very limited with the amount of treatment and care that we can actually give this lady with a view to improving the way she is now. So I think she is a lady who is going to need long-term hospital care. And that's a combination of both sort of physical and social problems really. Because I must admit she is a difficult lady to look after and I really don't think he would be able to cope at all with her now. Em, and they were relying quite a lot on neighbours and that for support. Em, another lady we have in is, she's just come in actually, but she is a lady who's already in a home for the elderly outside of hospital care, a social services home.

S.B.: Uhuh.

L.S.: Again, it's a lady who's had a fall in the home, em, and hasn't been very well for two days and in fact she's actually developed a chest infection which might have been sparked off by the fall because she's been in bed since then.

S.B.: I see.

L.S.: Em, and in fact has not been eating and has just deteriorated over the last couple of days. The thing is with this lady I don't think she will go to a long-stay ward because once we've got her over her chest infection and got her back on her feet and mobile again she will go back to the home from where she came.

S.B.: You mentioned in relation to the first patient you thought you'd be limited in how much you could achieve. Is this a fairly common characteristic of these patients?

L.S.: Em, not always, no I wouldn't say, it depends really on the medical condition or whatever it is that's brought them into hospital. One factor I do find is that on the, em, acute geriatric wards they tend to go for assessment first when we transfer them they sometimes go to an assessment ward and then on to a long-stay ward if that's what they require. But they have more, em, rehabilitation and physiotherapy facilities than we do on our ward. The reason is because they have their own staff that work on that department, where we have say one physiotherapist between four wards, em, so that they're not getting as much, em, walking and exercise and things that they do. So quite often you find that a lot of patients improve dramatically when they've spent a couple of weeks on a rehabilitation ward over there. So in fact sometimes it is the answer to send them to one of the rehabilitation wards, and then from there on to them being discharged and they may never need long-term care. So it doesn't always, that isn't always the problem really. Em, this is why I say we don't know with this particular lady. She may improve, although I'm pretty doubtful myself. She's a, mentally she's quite happy to sit in a chair and is very reluctant actually, em, to get up and be walked or have things explained, well 'you're going to get stiff if you sit in a chair', she doesn't want to know, she's quite happy just to doze off in the chair.

S.B.: When you refer a patient to the geriatrician you suggested that they're called in, what kind of things, or what kind of events or what is it about the patient that makes you decide you want to make the referral?

L.S.: Em, well social conditions are one if, em, we are running into problems because a patient is not able to cope at all, em, at home and is in unsuitable conditions, you know, perhaps, em, self neglect and this sort of thing, has no family or has a family who are not able to give us any assistance, that is one reason for a referral. It may be because of medical problems, em, depending on their condition, if they're going to need long-term care, a stroke for example.

S.B.: Uhuh.

L.S.: And they're going to be in for months, that's another reason. There are other medical problems that, em, we would refer them for, sometimes heart disorders, em, that again perhaps need long-term care, heart failures, em, they would go there but I must admit that a lot of them are due to social problems.

S.B.: Mm, so you wouldn't admit all, or refer all heart failures over the age of 70, necessarily to a geriatrician?

L.S.: No, no we don't. Actually we don't refer that many patients, em, we have a lot of elderly patients on our ward, em, we've got quite a few ladies now in their 80s that we haven't referred because either they've got a husband at home or whatever, we know that once we've got them over their medical illness they are going to be quite capable of caring for themselves or have family to support them when they go home. Em, the thing is I suppose in all areas of this country, waiting lists for alternative accommodation are tremendously long, em, but I suppose it comes down to bed blocking. I mean it sounds a bit awful but on an acute ward if you've got somebody who's maybe going to need eight months or more care while they're just waiting for a placement they're better where they are going to get more rehabilitation or whatever. But it may come down in fact, that they don't need the

	alternative accommodation that we are trying to arrange for them. Perhaps if they've been in one of the wards over there for a few months they might be able to rehabilitate them so that they do go back to their own homes for a while, maybe still pending alternative accommodation depending on how well that they've progressed. Em, but we don't refer, you know, every elderly patient.
S.B.:	Some of the ones you mentioned then who may be over 80 and have a heart failure or a similar condition, would you call them geriatrics? Would you refer to them as that, if you were discussing them?
L.S.:	Em, no. When we're talking amongst ourselves actually we tend even, I've talked to you about you know say geriatrics, but nursing staff, I don't know whether it's just now or, we tend not to refer to them as geriatric patients, em. We tend to say they've been referred to the geriatric clinic.
S.B.:	Uhuh.
L.S.:	Em, but we wouldn't sort of, when we're giving a report, refer to them as geriatrics, no, we tend to say they've been referred to the geriatric unit and then that's it, yes.

APPENDIX 2

(From the transcripts of the interviews recorded on Audio-cassette 1.
Presenter: Senga Bond, interviewee: Lynn Sadler.)

CONCERN WITH IMAGE

L.S.: Purely because the coronary care unit only has six beds and they cannot cater for every patient who's had a myocardial infarction and it's just unfortunate that they think that the younger people should have the closer observation from direct monitoring. Em, that doesn't always follow, if we've had a patient who's been 70 plus who perhaps develops arythmia.

S.B.: Yes.

L.S.: Em, and they do have a bed in the coronary care unit then they will admit that patient, but the unfortunate thing is, if they then get somebody of 28, 30 who's had a myocardial infarction then the older patients are moved out to accommodate the under 70s. It works quite well but, you know, I don't think it's ever been a great problem of the age cut-off, but the reason is they just couldn't cope with every patient.

L.S.: Now if we've got somebody who's maybe 70 and who just needs rehabilitation with a view to going home but perhaps needs to be in hospital a few more weeks, em, we'll refer them to the consultant who is in charge of that area. And likewise, if we have somebody who is from poor social circumstances who is not going to be able to cope on their own who really doesn't warrant a hospital admission long term then again the consultant actually from that area comes and assesses them for the ward. So in fact they assess the patient rather than us, the consultant comes across and sees them whilst they're still on my ward and allocates the ward that he would like them to go to and it's worked on that basis.

S.B.: So it's the geriatric consultant.

L.S.: That's right, yes.

S.B.: What, what kind of things would suggest that you would refer a patient for this consultation, because obviously it's a two way (L.S.: yes) thing. You suggest they come and see them. (L.S.: Yes.) With a view perhaps to making a decision.

L.S.: That's right. They also have a day hospital, a geriatric day hospital, so if for instance we have somebody, we cover quite a wide variety you see. It may be sort of things such as a cerebral tumour, it could be strokes, it could be cardiac problems, respiratory problems. Em, if we feel in fact that they could cope at home, they may be living with daughters, sons, but that they do need some relief or do need some hospital supervision but it doesn't need to be full term, we discharge them home and perhaps they come back to the day hospital two or three times a week, once a week.

S.B.: Yes.

L.S.: In that way they are getting some supervision from the hospital so that if things start to break down at home we know about them directly. Em, other things, em, we may get somebody in who is a stroke who is progressing very well but needs more rehabilitation so that the consultant might feel in fact that they are going to benefit

	from hospital admission for a couple of weeks, particularly with a view to daily living assessment because they have kitchens and things over there where they can actually be seen to how they're going to cope in household activities before being discharged, so they may in fact, they may go over there for a period of assessment for a week before being discharged.
S.B.:	Yes, yes.
L.S.:	But as I said if you get somebody with poor social circumstances or who is going not going to cope at all then they're the patients who would go on for longer care.
S.B.:	You mentioned in relation to the first patient you thought you'd be limited in how much you could achieve. Is this a fairly common characteristic of these patients?
L.S.:	Em, not always, no I wouldn't say, it depends really on the medical condition or whatever it is that's brought them into hospital. One factor I do find is that on the, em, acute geriatric wards they tend to go for assessment first when we transfer them they sometimes go to an assessment ward and then on to a long-stay ward if that's what they require. But they have more, em, rehabilitation and physiotherapy facilities than we do on our ward. The reason is because they have their own staff that work on that department, where we have say one physiotherapist between four wards, em, so that they're not getting as much, em, walking and exercise and things that they do. So quite often you find that a lot of patients improve dramatically when they've spent a couple of weeks on a rehabilitation ward over there. So in fact sometimes it is the answer to send them to one of the rehabilitation wards, and then from there on to them being discharged and they may never need long-term care. So it doesn't always, that isn't always the problem really. Em, this is why I say we don't know with this particular lady. She may improve, although I'm pretty doubtful myself. She's a, mentally she's quite happy to sit in a chair and is very reluctant actually, em, to get up and be walked or have things explained, well 'you're going to get stiff if you sit in a chair', she doesn't want to know, she's quite happy just to doze off in a chair.
S.B.:	When you refer a patient to the geriatrician you suggested that they're called in, what kind of things, or what kind of events or what is it about the patient that makes you decide you want to make the referral?
L.S.:	Em, well social conditions are one if, em, we are running into problems because a patient is not able to cope at all, em, at home and is in unsuitable conditions, you know, perhaps, em, self neglect and this sort of thing, has no family or has a family who are not able to give us any assistance, that is one reason for a referral. It may be because of medical problems, em, depending on their condition, if they're going to need long-term care, a stroke for example.
L.S.:	She was a very intelligent lady, em, she'd been a semi-professional flower arranger, em, and it was a combined discussion it wasn't just between nurses and doctors but it was with physiotherapists and the occupational therapist. And in fact the geriatric consultant himself felt that one of his long-stay wards would not be the answer for this particular patient.

UNIT 19/20 ANALYSIS OF STRUCTURED DATA

Prepared for the Course Team by Judith Calder

CONTENTS

Associated study materials		40
1	**Introduction**	41
	1.1 Different kinds of data	42
2	**Approaches to analysis**	44
	2.1 Looking at variables	44
	2.2 Two types of statistics	46
3	**Descriptive measures**	46
	3.1 Measures of central tendency	46
	3.2 Measures of spread	49
	3.3 Measures of location	50
4	**Inferential statistics**	52
	4.1 Types of error	52
	4.2 Chi-square	55
	4.3 z and t tests	63
	4.4 Analysis of variance	65
5	**Correlation and regression**	69
	5.1 Correlation coefficients	69
	5.2 Simple linear regression	73
6	**Multivariate analyses**	76
	6.1 Tabular techniques	76
	Extended example	77
	6.2 More on analysis of variance	80
	6.3 Regression techniques	83
	6.4 Related multivariate approaches	87
	Log-linear analysis	87
	Discriminant analysis	88
	6.5 Factor analysis	90
7	**Final comments**	92
Answers to activities		92
Further reading		99
References		99
Acknowledgements		99

ASSOCIATED STUDY MATERIALS

Offprints Booklet 4, 'How non-volatile is brainpower?', *Electronics World and Wireless World*.

Offprints Booklet 4, 'How long does education last? Very long term retention of cognitive psychology', by Gillian Cohen, Nicola Stanhope and Martin Conway.

Offprints Booklet 4, 'Age differences in the retention of knowledge by young and elderly students', by Gillian Cohen, Nicola Stanhope and Martin Conway.

Statistics Handbook

In addition you will need the NUMERACY computer-assisted learning disk and also use of FRAMEWORK is recommended.

At the end of the unit there is an extended exercise (Activity 15) to help prepare you for TMA 07. For this you will need:

Audio-cassette programme 'Analysing structured data',

Audio-visual Handbook, and

OUSTATS disk and RECON data-file on the computer.

1 INTRODUCTION

By this stage in the course, you are probably wondering just how much of what has been covered you will actually remember, and for how long. You may be concerned about your recall of issues and facts, not just for the exams, but if you want to go on and use the knowledge and understanding gained from studying the course. One variable which is often assumed to affect people's memory and powers of recall is their age. During the 1980s a small group of academics at the Open University carried out research on memory, recall, and the effects of age on the retention of knowledge over time. Associated with this unit is a set of three readings which report some of their work. Although the readings are all reports of the same research study, they handle the findings in rather different ways. In this unit we will be drawing on these readings as examples of the way in which research which has produced structured data can be reported. The particular aspect of the methodology on which we are focusing is data analysis. You may be familiar with Mark Twain's aphorism about 'lies, damned lies and statistics'. By finding out what form of analysis uses what type of statistic and, importantly, how they might be interpreted, you will be able to 'give the lie' to this somewhat jaundiced view of a very useful and much misunderstood set of tools. Do not forget that this unit is seen as *two* weeks' work, including the cassette-led exercise at the end, so you should have plenty of time to get to grips with some of the more difficult concepts which are introduced.

In presenting the ideas and techniques of statistics I have tried, as far as possible, to keep the mathematical equations *out* of the main text. Instead they are supplied in boxes labelled 'Stats Pieces'. It is worth trying to read them as they do add to your understanding of the concepts. A useful way of approaching this unit might be to read it once, fairly quickly, doing the activities but ignoring the Stats Pieces; then go back over it and see what a reading of the Stats Pieces can add to your understanding.

READING AND ACTIVITY 1

Scan the three readings associated with this unit reproduced in Offprints Booklet 4, making notes on the major similarities and differences between the articles in the way the data are presented and the terms in which they are discussed. Make a note of those parts you find particularly difficult to handle or interpret. Do not spend more than about 20 minutes on this activity.

At the end of this unit you will be asked to go back over your notes to see if any of the problems have been clarified.

The three readings are:

1 'How non-volatile is brainpower?', *Electronics World and Wireless World*.

2 'How long does education last? Very long term retention of cognitive psychology', by G. Cohen, N. Stanhope and M. Conway.

3 'Age differences in the retention of knowledge by young and elderly students', by G. Cohen, N. Stanhope and M. Conway.

As you will have noticed, each of the readings is written for a different audience. The reports differ in the amount and type of methodological and statistical detail which they present to the reader. The report written for the non-specialist audience has little technical detail, whereas those written for professional peers contain a great deal. It is not necessary, however, to be able to carry out or to have a detailed knowledge of the mechanics of all statistical procedures in order to be able to interpret their appropriateness and importance. Just as you can be a perfectly competent driver without understanding the detailed workings of the combustion engine or hydraulic systems, so it is possible to read and use the output from statistical analyses without having a detailed knowledge of the mathematics which underlie them.

In a similar way, the rapid spread of computers and the accompanying increase in their memory and processing power now means that researchers are able to carry out data analyses involving long and complex formulae without actually knowing what the formulae are and without having to get directly involved in any of the calculations. This has both advantages and disadvantages. The power of computers has enabled researchers to start using very sophisticated techniques which would previously not have been feasible. At the same time, however, it means that it is very easy for techniques to be used inappropriately. Advanced techniques used on the wrong sort of data will produce output from the computer which looks impressive but which is meaningless.

After having worked through this unit you should not only be in a position to read and understand a wider range of research papers and reports, but you should also be able to tell when conclusions may be suspect because of the inappropriate use of a particular form of analysis.

1.1 DIFFERENT KINDS OF DATA

Data can be categorized into two *types*. Some data such as time, temperature and length are examples of data which are continuous; that is, they can take values *between* whole numbers. So it is meaningful to say that a person is 36.33 years old for example. Other data are only meaningful as whole numbers. In spite of the predilection of newspapers for such families, you cannot have 2.4 children, for example! So these data, which have gaps between them rather than running in a continuous range, are known as discrete data. Examples of discrete and continuous data are shown in Table 1.

Table 1 Types of data and levels of measurement

Level of measurement	Discrete data	Continuous data
Nominal	Gender	—
	Name of town	
	Exam subjects	
Ordinal	Birth position in family	—
	Exam grades	
Interval	Exam scores	Temperature
Ratio	Family size	Income
	Number of exam passes	Age

The amount of information which data may give can vary considerably, and we can also categorize them by the kinds of information they yield and the kinds of calculations that can be done with them. In the first column of Table 1 you can see four *levels of measurement* listed. Nominal data (sometimes known as *categorical data* for obvious reasons) give the least information, recording merely the name of the group or category to which an individual or item belongs. Occupational categories like miners, farmers, home helps, sheet metal workers, are a typical example of nominal data.

Ordinal data (sometimes called *ranked data*) indicate the rank order that someone or something holds, but give no indication of distance between ranks. The fact that a child may be the second child in a family reveals nothing about distance in age from the older sibling; a youngster could be (say) 14 months or 14 years younger than their older sibling and still be the second child in the family. Football league tables, social class groupings and GCSE grades are all examples of ordinal groupings. If one person has a GCSE grade C and another has a GCSE grade D, you know that the C grade is higher than the D grade, but not by how much. Rating scales which use classifications like 'very important', 'fairly important', 'not very important', 'not at all important', produce ordinal data.

In contrast, *interval data* may be used to calculate how far apart measures are — there are equal intervals or equal distances between each of the measures on the scale. However, with interval data there is no *absolute* zero point. Thus it is not possible to divide or to multiply one score by another. Measurements of temperature are one example given of interval data, where a temperature of 40°C cannot be divided by a temperature of 20°C to claim that 40°C is twice as hot as 20°C. There is what is *called* a zero, at 0°C, but this is merely a point of reference against which other temperature measures can be set. Someone who scored 80 per cent in an exam, will not necessarily be twice as good or know twice as much as someone who achieved a score of 40 per cent. In other words, you can specify the distance between the two data points, but not their worth in relation to each other.

Finally, where we have *ratio data*, we can draw conclusions about the *relative size or* worth of the data (hence the term 'ratio'). For example, a youngster with six GCSE grade C passes will have twice as many as someone with three grade C passes. A person's income, regardless of the units in which it is measured, can be expressed as a ratio of someone else's. So, for example, we can say that people earning £30,000 have twice as much as people earning £15,000.

It will be apparent from these examples that it can sometimes be quite difficult to identify correctly the type of data that is being investigated. Statisticians have pointed out that, strictly speaking, although data such as intelligence, aptitude and personality tests have numerical scores attached to them, they are only ordinal data. They cannot be ratio data because there is no real or absolute zero. Nor can they be interval data because there is no guarantee that the values are equidistant. However, they do fulfil the requirements of ordinal data by indicating the rank order position of individuals. For example, no one can have a zero intelligence. Not only that, but the apparent distances between two data points may not reflect their real difference. Is the difference in IQ between 135 and 145 the same as the difference between an IQ of 65 and 75? Thus the criterion for ratio data, of having a true and meaningful zero, is not met, and it is arguable as to whether the criterion for interval data, of having equal distances on a measured scale, is met either. This last point is a weakness often found in data which are treated as interval. For example, rating scales usually have numbers attached to them which researchers tend to treat as if they were equidistant. For example:

Very important	1
Fairly important	2
Not very important	3 — ordinal
Not at all important	4

The problem is that the 'real' distance between the ratings numbered 3 and 4 for a respondent may be much greater than the distance they perceive between the items numbered 1 and 2. The 'real' distances between each of the ratings may also vary from person to person. In theory, therefore, such data should be treated as ordinal data. Most researchers take a pragmatic approach, however, and continue with the practice of treating ratings and psychological tests as interval data.

One way of dealing with data which are difficult to 'type' correctly is through the use of *models*. Scientists use models of weather systems to study the relationships between different factors in order to understand better what the contributory factors are. In the same way, statisticians produce statistical models based on their current understanding of a problem. When they do not quite work as expected, they modify some of their assumptions. If the assumption of an interval scale does not work, then further analyses can be carried out on the assumption of an ordinal scale. Over the years, reviews of the statistical evidence suggest that the assumption of equality of equal intervals within rating scales is justified. But where such assumptions are made, there is always the *possibility* of misinterpretation of the data. The important point is to be clear always that there are different types of data, and that this will affect the type of analyses which can be used on them.

ACTIVITY 2

See if you can think of four clear examples of each kind of data (nominal, ordinal, interval and ratio), from the three readings associated with this unit in Offprints Booklet 4 or from elsewhere. Take note of any kind of data you find difficult to classify.

My answers to activities are at the end of the unit.

2 APPROACHES TO ANALYSIS

2.1 LOOKING AT VARIABLES

We have been discussing the fact that the level and type of data you are dealing with can have a considerable influence on the type of analysis you are able to undertake. A number of other criteria also play a key role in determining the approach which is used for the analysis; for example, the amount and type of units of analysis, the number of variables, the research design, the sample design and sample size, and, most importantly, the research question(s).

Remember that the aim of analysis is to get information and draw conclusions from the data which have been collected. In the piece of research being reported in the readings, there were 373 respondents. The researchers had to look at the results of a questionnaire and five different memory tests for each of these respondents and then draw general conclusions from them. Many quantitative studies in education and the social sciences are much larger than this, involving samples of thousands, with questionnaires of considerable length which collect data about hundreds of attributes and variables. In order to draw conclusions from the data collected it is necessary to look for patterns in the data, to summarize and reduce the data and to look for relationships between different variables.

In general, one of the key points which must be established as early as possible is which of the variables are seen as being dependent and which as independent. A variable is termed *independent* if, for a particular research question, it is hypothesized as being the cause of some effect on a *dependent* variable. For example, if we hypothesize that a person's income is affected by their gender, then, for this research question, income would be the dependent variable and gender the independent variable. The independent variable is always the antecedent and the dependent variable the consequent. It would never be hypothesized that someone's gender was in some way influenced by their income, for example! So in the question addressed in the third reading associated with this unit (Cohen *et al.*, 1992b) it is concluded that retention of knowledge from an undergraduate degree course in cognitive psychology (the dependent variable) is affected by the retention interval (independent variable) and the grade originally achieved (independent variable) (see Figure 1).

UNIT 19/20 ANALYSIS OF STRUCTURED DATA

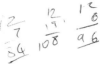

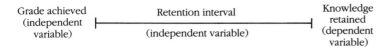

Time

Figure 1 *The causal sequence*

Table 2 Subject totals and means by retention interval for age, grade and contact

RI in months	Subject totals		Age at retrieval		Grade		Contact	
	T	%	M	SD	M	SD	M	SD
3	33	8.8	39.6	8.1	2.5	.834	1.88	.331
15	37	9.9	39.8	8.9	2.5	.650	1.65	.484
27	35	9.4	45.5	10.1	2.7	1.01	1.57	.502
39	25	6.7	46.7	11.1	2.8	.913	1.60	.500
41	42	11.3	46.8	9.4	2.8	.881	1.69	.468
53	48	12.9	48.5	10.1	2.5	.849	1.60	.494
65	28	7.5	52.9	8.7	2.8	.803	1.68	.476
77	27	7.2	54.4	11.6	3.0	.898	1.78	.424
89	27	7.2	55.7	10.0	2.9	.759	1.63	.492
101	23	6.2	52.6	10.7	2.4	.988	1.57	.507
113	18	4.8	53.3	11.9	2.8	.707	1.89	.323
125	30	8.1	58.9	9.6	2.4	.817	1.63	.490

RI = retention interval; T = total; M = mean; and SD = standard deviation.
Contact refers to ratings of contact with course material with the exception of research methods.
Note: the authors draw the attention of readers to the fact that 'the spacing of RIs is not equal, and this is because testing was conducted in two waves some months apart'.
(Source: Conway et al., 1991, p.398, Table 1)

Now look at Table 2, reproduced from Conway *et al.* (1991), which is another report from the same research team. When you read research articles or reports always check what the symbols stand for in case they are being used in a way with which you are not familiar. You will have noted in Table 2 that M and SD are used as the symbols for the mean and standard deviation, rather than the more usual $\bar{x}$ and s. In this unit, we will normally stay with the convention detailed in the Statistics Handbook. The data in Table 2 clearly are already summarized. The RI column (RI stands for retention interval) shows how long it was between the student studying the course and being tested, while going down the next column (T for total) we can see how many former students last studied the psychology course 3 months ago, 15 months ago, 27 months ago, and so on. The information about the retention intervals of the former students has been *grouped* into frequencies for each of the retention intervals, so the researchers are here dealing with only twelve measures rather than the 373 they started with. The rest of the table similarly summarizes information about the former students. Reading across the table this time, you can see that for the 33 students who last studied psychology 3 months prior to testing, their mean age (M) at the time of the study was 39.6 years, and the standard deviation (SD) about the mean age for that group of 33 people was 8.1 years. Moving further along the same line, we read that the mean grade for their psychology courses achieved by this group of former students was 2.5 (remember that 2 is the code for an upper second and 3 the code for a lower second class degree) with a standard deviation of 0.834, and, further along, that the mean contact level for this group was 1.88. Again this score can only be interpreted if you know that contact was coded either as 1 for a considerable amount of post-course contact with psychology, or 2 for only a little or no further contact with the field after completing the course. These statistics, then, are *describing* the data which has been collected.

2.2 TWO TYPES OF STATISTICS

In the table at which we have been looking, no hypotheses are being tested nor inferences drawn about a wider population. Such statistics, which focus on the description of data presented, are known as *descriptive statistics*. In contrast, *inferential statistics* are used in order to draw conclusions about a wider population from sample data and to examine differences, similarities and relationships between different variables. There are two aspects to inferential statistics.

1. The first concerns the making of inferences about populations from data drawn from samples. For example, if 29 per cent of our *sample* listen to a certain radio programme, then we use that information to make an inference about the percentage of our *population* who listen to that radio programme. Statistical techniques are used to estimate the range within which the population parameters are likely to lie, given the sample statistics. (You may remember this being discussed in Unit 8.)

2. The second aspect comes from the testing of hypotheses or the study of relationships. Here the emphasis is on hypotheses about the data being studied. In the research reported in the readings, we can see that the researchers have tested a number of hypotheses about the relationship between age, retention interval and amount and quality of recall. Statistical techniques are used to assess how likely it is that the observed difference or relationship could arise by chance alone if the same difference was not to be found in the population from which the sample was drawn.

3 DESCRIPTIVE MEASURES

In Table 2 several different kinds of descriptive statistics were used. We saw frequency scores, percentages, means and standard deviations referred to. You have met these already in Units 8 and 16. Let us just spend a moment looking at each one of these and revise the concepts introduced there. First, the frequency scores for the retention intervals can be plotted as a graph. When the points are joined together, we have a *distribution* of retention interval frequencies from 3 months to 125 months (see Figure 2).

To summarize and describe the distribution in Figure 2 three pieces of information are needed. First, we need information about what is called the *central tendency* in order to see where the central values or 'typical' values are located. Secondly, we need information about the variability or spread among the values of the variable. Thirdly, we need information about the location of individual values relative to the other values in the distribution.

3.1 MEASURES OF CENTRAL TENDENCY

You will recall that the three measures of central tendency are the mean, median and mode. The mean is simply the average of all the data. The median is the middle value of the ordered data, i.e. when the data are arranged from the

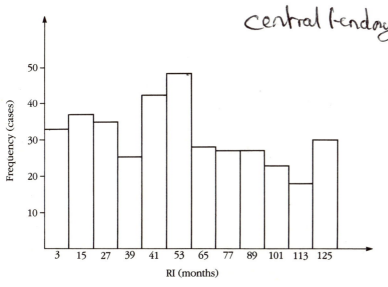

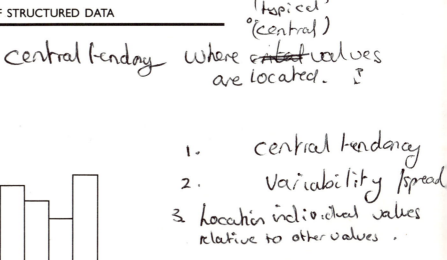

Figure 2 *Distribution of retention interval frequencies*
(Source: based on Conway et al., 1991, Table 1)

smallest up to the largest, or vice versa. The mode is the value which is most common in the data set (hence the link with the now rather old fashioned word 'modish'). As you can see in Figure 3, if the distribution is a normal distribution, the mean, median and mode will be the same. If the distribution is *skewed* — if it is not symmetrical — they will have different values (see Figure 4).

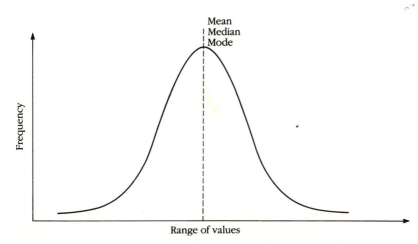

Figure 3 *Normal distribution*

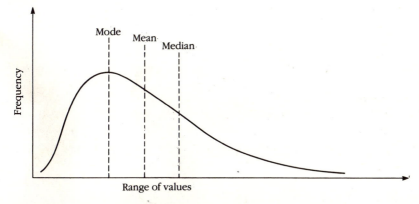

Figure 4 *Skewed distribution*

STATS PIECE 1: MEAN, MEDIAN AND MODE

Mean

For a data set of N different measures

$$x_1, x_2, x_3, \ldots, x_i, \ldots, x_N$$

the mean is

$$\bar{x} = \frac{x_1 + x_2 + \ldots + x_N}{N}$$

$$= \frac{\sum x_i}{N}$$

where Σ (sigma) is a symbol which means 'the sum of'.

Median

The median is the value of the centre of the ordered data set.

So if N is odd:

$$\text{median} = \text{the value of the } \frac{N+1}{2}\text{th data value.}$$

If N is even:

median = the average of the two central data values.

For example, a data set of students' ages might be:

21 23 23 28 30 35 35 35 42 42 44 58 63 67 71

There are fifteen pieces of data, so the median is the

$$\frac{15+1}{2} = \text{8th data value} = 35 \text{ years.}$$

If there were fourteen pieces of data, e.g.

23 23 28 30 35 35 35 42 42 44 58 63 67 71

then the median would be the average of the two central values:

$$\frac{35+42}{2} = \frac{77}{2} = 38.5 \text{ years.}$$

Mode

The mode is the most frequent or most common value. In the example above, with fifteen pieces of data, all the values occur once only with the exception of 23, 35 and 42. Both 23 and 42 occur twice, and 35 occurs three times. The modal age would therefore be 35 years.

3.2 MEASURES OF SPREAD

As Figure 5 shows, however, it is quite possible to have two distributions with the same mean, but with very different distributions of values. The spread, or the variability, of the distribution for (b) is much greater than that for (a). A second piece of information is therefore needed to summarize and describe a distribution: namely, some measure of its spread or variability. The simplest measure for doing this is to look at the *range* of the data scores or measures. In the research reported in the readings the retention interval ranges from 3 months to 125 months, a range of 122 months. This figure gives quite a good indication of the actual spread of the data, because the frequencies are relatively even. However, if we were looking at the age of the former students, and there was one very elderly person of, say, 90 years with everyone else being under the age of 65 years, then the range of ages would not be a good indicator of spread because of the distortion introduced by the extreme case. (These extreme cases are often referred to as *outliers*.) Any extreme cases will mean that the range over-estimates the spread of the data. The *interquartile range*, which looks only at the middle 50 per cent of the distribution, is a better indicator, and it is frequently used as an indicator in economics. However, the most useful and most powerful indicator of spread is the *standard deviation*.

STATS PIECE 2: STANDARD DEVIATION

For a sample data set of *n* different measures:

$$x_1, x_2, \ldots, x_n$$

the variance is

$$s^2 = \frac{(x_1 - \bar{x})^2 + (x_2 - \bar{x})^2 + \ldots + (x_i - \bar{x})^2 + \ldots + (x_n - \bar{x})^2}{n - 1}$$

$$= \frac{\Sigma(x_i - \bar{x})^2}{n - 1}$$

hence the standard deviation is

$$s = \sqrt{\frac{\Sigma(x_i - \bar{x})^2}{n - 1}}.$$

You will recall from Unit 8 that the standard deviation will be small where the data cluster closely around the mean, and where the standard deviation is large, it is because the data are spread out. So, for example, in Figure 5 (b) will have a larger standard deviation than (a).

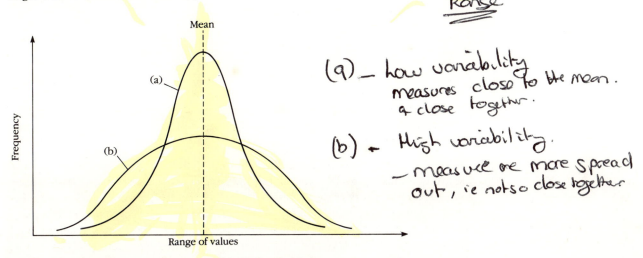

Figure 5 (a) Low variability and (b) high variability

ACTIVITY 3

Look at the 'age at retrieval' column in Table 2 and identify which RI groups have the greatest differences in the spread of ages as measured by the standard deviations of their mean ages.

3.3 MEASURES OF LOCATION

In social and economic research, the different variables which comprise a data set are often measured in different units: for example, time, attitude ratings, income and occupation. In the research reported in the readings, the units used were months and years (RI and age), and grades and rating scores (interest). In order to make comparisons between distributions using different measures, the measurements have to be transformed in order that they can all be located on one common scale. Even simple operations like addition or multiplication are not possible on data which are not comparable because they are measured in different units. One common way of achieving this is to use *percentages*, as we saw in Units 6 and 16. Notice that in the extract from the third reading, reproduced as Table 3, the data are presented in this form, enabling easy comparisons to be made between the different sub-groups.

Table 3 Differences by age in grade and interest scores

(a) Percentages of young, middle-aged and elderly subjects distributed across grades

Age	Grade				Mean
	1 (high)	2	3	4 (low)	
Young	14	37	42	7	2.43
Middle-aged	6	29	48	17	2.77
Elderly	8	18	48	26	2.92

(b) Percentages of young, middle-aged and elderly subjects distributed across different levels of interest

Age	Interest			Mean
	1 (high)	2	3 (low)	
Young	44	46	10	1.66
Middle-aged	52	41	7	1.55
Elderly	66	33	1	1.36

Note: in both these tables the data have been percentaged *across* each row.
(Source: Cohen et al., 1992b, Tables 1b and 1c)

The use of percentages in this way means that it is very easy to see any differences, within each table, between the distribution of grades and of interest for the different age groups.

The third reading, 'Age differences in the retention of knowledge by young and elderly students', also includes a set of three *contingency* tables. Contingency tables are any form of table in which the cell entries show the frequencies, or the proportions or percentages based on frequencies. As in Unit 16, you can have three- or even four-variable contingency tables, though they are sometimes difficult to interpret. Table 4 has two variables, age and retention interval. Age is broken into three categories and retention interval into six groupings, displayed as three rows and six columns, and would therefore be known as a three by six contingency table. All three of the contingency tables in the third reading are two-way tables because they look at two variables at a time.

Table 4 Percentages of young, middle-aged and elderly subjects distributed across retention intervals

Age	Retention intervals in years					
	0.25–2	3–4	5–6	7–8	9–10	11–12
Young	41	22	23	7	4	3
Middle-aged	12	15	29	18	14	12
Elderly	4	11	12	16	26	30

(Source: Cohen et al., 1992b, Table 1a)

ACTIVITY 4

What does Table 4 tell us — how are we to interpret it? How might it be made more interpretable?

Another way of handling this issue is through the use of units based on standard deviations, known as *standard scores* or *z-scores*. These units are used most frequently in the analysis of educational and psychological tests. Remember that the standard deviation measures the spread of a group of data, such as scores, by examining the distance of the individual scores from the mean. The *z*-score simply transforms each score into the number of standard deviations or fractions of standard deviations it is away from the mean. A key feature of *z* is that by transforming any measure from a distribution into a *z*-score, it is possible to say how likely it is that a particular *z*-score will lie between certain limits or how far from the mean an observation is located. This means that where researchers have to deal with estimates of population data or with sample data, they are able to assign probabilities through the use of *z*. Thus *z* transformations form one of the basic building blocks in inferential statistics.

STATS PIECE 3: z-SCORES

$$z = \frac{x - \bar{x}}{s}$$

where s is the standard deviation.

For example, suppose in the research reported in the readings we had a former student who had finished her studies 3 months prior to the research and whose age at the time of the study was 52 years. Then from row 1 of Table 2 we could take the additional information ($\bar{x}$ and s) to calculate z.

Say

$x = 52.0$,

from Table 2

$\bar{x} = 39.6$

and

$s = 8.1$,

therefore using the formula the z-score for her age would be:

$$z = \frac{x - \bar{x}}{s} = \frac{52 - 39.6}{8.1}$$

$$= +1.53.$$

So the student would have a z-score of +1.53 for her age. In other words the z-score tells us that her age is 1.53 standard deviations above the group mean.

Descriptive statistics are the most widely used measures in research reports and papers. We have discussed the three major measures of central tendency, measures of variability and measures of location which are used in descriptive statistics. Each of them summarizes the set of data it is describing in a different way. Remember that although descriptive statistics comprise these simple measures, they also underpin what are called inferential statistics.

ACTIVITY 5

Read the following two quotes taken from the extracts in Offprints Booklet 4 and comment on the descriptive statistics that are mentioned.

> Results published in *The Psychologist* ... show that even very recent graduates can rarely remember more than about 70 per cent of the factual data they were taught.
>
> (*Electronics World and Wireless World*, 1992)
>
> In the fact verification test, scores initially averaged around 70%. Memory for specific facts declined to 65 per cent after three years. Although performance at longer retention intervals was somewhat variable, there was no significant decline.
>
> (Cohen et al., 1992a)

4 INFERENTIAL STATISTICS

You will recall that earlier in the unit you were briefly introduced to the two aspects of inferential statistics: hypothesis testing, and estimation of population parameters from sample data (Section 2.2). As you will see in the next section, the same measure or test is often used for both purposes. Remember that inferential statistics are about generalizing from the evidence available. Researchers can either generalize from the sample to the population, as you saw in Unit 8, or they can test hypotheses about relationships or differences in the population, using the data from the sample. Either way, because the results are based on samples, they will be subject to sampling error. With either type of conclusion, inferential statistics enables you to say with what level of uncertainty the findings should be treated.

4.1 TYPES OF ERROR

Not surprisingly, a hypothesis has to be expressed in statistical terms before it can be tested. But it always has to be tested against some alternative. In fact you can never actually prove statistically that a hypothesis is right. You can only show either that it should be rejected or that it should not be rejected. (Hence the difficulty of proving statistically that there is an association between lung cancer and smoking, or between radiation and childhood leukaemia.) The actual formulation of the hypothesis is therefore very important.

Suppose a large institution has an equal opportunities target for its staffing profile. Their aim is 5 per cent of employees who could be classified as people with physical disabilities. The question is whether this target has been attained or whether further action needs to be taken to achieve it. A small sample study involving 140 staff is carried out which gives a figure of 2.7 per cent of staff who could be categorized as people with physical disabilities. The sample data suggests that the target has not been reached. However, it might be argued that the figure of 2.7 per cent of staff had emerged by chance because of the particular sample which was selected, and that the target figure for the staff as a whole had actually been reached. For this sort of problem, two hypotheses have to be presented. The researchers form what is known as the *null* hypothesis (written as H_0), which says that the target has been reached. That is, they propose there is no significant difference between the sample figure and the target figure. The alternative hypothesis H_a is that the target has not been reached. The null hypothesis is always the one which is actually tested. The researchers can then show either that the null hypothesis should be rejected and that therefore there is a likelihood that the target has not been reached, or that the null hypothesis is not rejected and that therefore it is likely that the target *has* been reached.

When researchers are drawing conclusions from a sample, there is the danger of two different types of incorrect conclusions being drawn from the evidence available. The null hypothesis may be rejected when it is true (so in the example above, scarce resources may be spent unnecessarily in continuing to try to reach the target) or the null hypothesis may not be rejected when in fact it is false (i.e. it is assumed that the target has been reached when in fact it has not).

These two types of error are referred to as Type 1 and Type 2 errors.

- If the null hypothesis H_0 is rejected when in fact it is true, then you have a Type 1 error.

- If the null hypothesis H_0 is not rejected when in fact it is false, then you have a Type 2 error.

Whenever a hypothesis is being tested, the probability that either of these errors will occur can be calculated. The probability of a Type 1 error, i.e. rejecting H_0 when it is true, is written as α. The probability of a Type 2 error, i.e. not rejecting H_0 when it is false, is written as β. Table 5 shows a summary of the situation.

Table 5 Types of error

Real situation	Conclusion drawn from test	
	reject H_0	do not reject H_0
H_0 true	Type 1 error $p = \alpha$	correct
H_0 false	correct[a]	Type 2 error $p = \beta$

[a] The probability of achieving the appropriate conclusion when the null hypothesis H_0 is false, that is, of correctly rejecting H_0 when it is false, is known as the *power* of a statistical test. This term is used frequently in research and statistical literature.

Alpha, or α, the Type 1 error, is also known as the *significance level*. In order to carry out a test on the hypothesis, the researchers have to decide what level they wish to set α at. The job of the hypothesis test then is to calculate the probability that the test statistic lies within a range which is fixed by the level the researchers selected for α (see Figure 6 on next page). The shaded *area* in Figure 6 shows the significance level α.

If the test statistic is found to lie outside the range set, then H_0 would be rejected. *But*, in reality one of two things could have occurred. Either H_0 was outside the limits because H_0 was actually false, or it was actually true but was outside because the test involves the use of sample data, and sample estimates will always

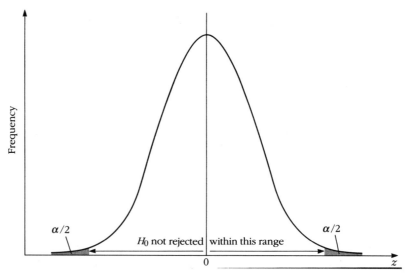

Figure 6 *Standard normal distribution. Each shaded area represents $\alpha/2$ so both together represent α*

carry a small but known probability of being an extreme measure. This you will now recognize would be a Type 1 error. Similarly if the statistic falls inside the limits, then the null hypothesis would not be rejected. However, here there is still a possibility that H_0 is actually false and that the statistic fell within these limits by chance. This would be a Type 2 error.

Note that for the Type 2 error, the term 'not rejected' rather than 'accepted' is used. The distinction between the terms 'not rejecting' and 'accepting' a hypothesis is an important one in research.

So how is α determined? At the beginning of the example, it was explained that the job of the hypothesis test is to calculate the probability that the null hypothesis H_0 can safely be rejected, and what counts as 'safe' is determined by the level the researchers selected for α. If α is minimized, then β is maximized. Conversely if β is minimized, then α is maximized. The issue of whether researchers should minimize the Type 1 error or the Type 2 error depends very much on the problem being investigated. In some instances, a Type 2 error can have very serious effects. For example: say the null hypothesis H_0 was that the attempted suicide rate was not increasing. Then α would be the probability of rejecting H_0 when it was true. That is, the data suggested that an increase had occurred when this was not the case (= Type 1 error). And β would be the probability that the test suggested that there had not been an increase when in fact there had been one (= Type 2 error).

Clearly in dealing with such issues, the aim of researchers analysing the data would be to minimize as far as possible the probability of Type 2 errors. In contrast, other situations would be such that the researchers would want to minimize the probability of Type 1 errors. If there is no reason to expect any differences between the effects of either type of error, then α is usually fixed at 0.05. An α of 0.05 means that there are five chances in 100 of making a Type 1 error, with H_0 being wrongly rejected when it is true. Similarly an α of 0.001 means there is only one chance in 1,000 of making a Type 1 error. Unfortunately the smaller α is made, the larger is the probability of a Type 2 error. By convention researchers tend to set α equal to 0.05 (one chance in 20 of Type 1 error) or the more stringent 0.01 (one chance in 100), but where it is to be set must depend on the nature of the research problem.

ACTIVITY 6

Think of an example where the null hypothesis was such that researchers would want to minimize the possibility of Type 1 errors.

You may have remarked by now that there is no reference to either α or β in the three readings for this unit. The reason is that a measure called the *observed significance level* or *p value* is normally used to indicate the exact point at which H_0 is either rejected or not rejected. Again, the decision to reject or not to reject H_0 may be made by the researchers on the basis of the chosen value for α. If the *p* value is less than α, then H_0 is rejected. If the *p* value is greater than or equal to α, then H_0 is not rejected. So, for example, if α has been set at .05, and *p* is calculated to be .15, then H_0 would not be rejected (see Figure 7). Alternatively, rather than choosing a specific value for α, what often happens is that where $p < .01$ then H_0 is rejected, and where $p > .05$ then H_0 is not rejected. If *p* lies between .01 and .05 then the results are usually considered to be inconclusive.

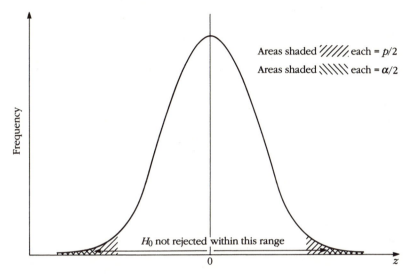

Figure 7 *Standard normal distribution. Remember that p and α are areas, so when p is bigger than the α which has been set it moves into the 'H_0 not rejected' zone.*

4.2 CHI-SQUARE

We have been talking about the errors that can occur when a null hypothesis is being tested. In the readings which accompany this unit, the researchers were investigating such hypotheses as whether there is any relationship between the grades a student achieves on a course and their age, or between their level of interest in the course and their age. So these are the sorts of hypotheses the researchers have in mind when they construct contingency tables from the research data.

Look again at the contingency tables reproduced as Tables 3 and 4 above. They are designed to reveal whether there is any association between age and grade achieved (Table 3a), age and interest (Table 3b) and age and retention interval (Table 4). In other words, the distribution of young, middle-aged and elderly subjects is examined across different levels of retention interval, different levels of grade achieved and different levels of interest. The researchers report that there is an association between age and all three variables. They report this in the third reading as follows.

> By χ^2 the distribution of age groups is significantly different for all these variables: RI (χ^2 (10) = 98.42, $p < .0001$); grade (χ^2 (6) = 18.40, $p < .005$); and interest (χ^2 (4) = 10.90, $p < .02$).
>
> (Cohen *et al.*, 1992b)

If you are a new reader of academic journals, the first word of advice on how to handle this piece of information is: don't panic! This statement is merely a succinct summary of some of the test results expressed in statistical terms. By unpacking the statement and examining each piece of information, we can interpret what the researchers are reporting about what the data reveals.

The χ^2 referred to in the paper is sometimes written as chi-square (pronounced ky-square as if it rhymes with 'why'-square), and is a key test used to establish whether or not the two variables of the contingency table (or cross-tabulation) are independent of each other. For example, if there is no association between age and grade, then you would expect the proportion of elderly former students who got high grades to be similar to the proportion of young former students getting high grades. The null hypothesis being tested, then, is that the frequencies or proportions found in the cells of the contingency table are what you would expect to find if there was no association. The chi-square test itself is based on the differences between the actual observed frequencies and the frequencies which would be expected if the null hypothesis were true.

STATS PIECE 4: CHI-SQUARE TEST

The formula used to test the hypothesis that the row and the column variables are independent is called the chi-square test, where

$$\chi^2 = \Sigma \frac{(O - E)^2}{E}.$$

The χ^2 test compares the observed frequency O in each table cell with the corresponding expected frequency E. Adding together all the resulting differences (or residuals) means that the value of chi-square depends on the number of rows and columns in the table. This means that the likelihood of a particular value of χ^2 occurring by chance will vary, depending on the number of rows and columns in the table. Special tables are available which enable researchers to look up this likelihood, or probability as it is termed (see the Statistics Handbook). More usually, the p value (discussed in Section 4.1) is calculated automatically when a statistical software package is used for the data analysis.

Let us look at the same extract that we looked at just now laid out slightly differently.

> By χ^2 the distribution of age groups is significantly different for all these variables:
>
> RI (χ^2 (10) = 98.42, p < .0001);
>
> grade (χ^2 (6) = 18.40, p < .005); and
>
> interest (χ^2 (4) = 10.90, p < .02).
>
> (Cohen *et al.*, 1992b)

In this extract from the reading we are given three figures, for the chi-square values of each of the three tables. These figures measure the differences between the frequencies which actually emerged or were observed in the research and the frequencies expected by chance. In order to interpret them we need to look at the rest of the information.

The number in parentheses after χ^2 in the extract refers to *degrees of freedom*: in this unit's text we normally use the initials *df*. This term simply means the number of independent terms in the table — that is, the opportunity for variation in the content of the cells, given that the row and column totals are fixed. For example, a 2 × 2 table (see Table 6), has only one degree of freedom. This is because once we know the row and column totals, only *one* figure in the body of the table is free to vary and we can work out all the rest by subtraction (i.e. the cells which are shaded). So only one figure in the table can come as any surprise.

UNIT 19/20 ANALYSIS OF STRUCTURED DATA

Table 6 Degrees of freedom for a 2 × 2 table

		Variable 1		Total
		1	2	
Variable 2	1	a	b	a + b
	2	c	d	c + d
Total		a + c	b + d	a + b + c + d

You can test this for yourselves by putting your own figures into cell *a* and into the row and column totals, and working out what the shaded cells should be. Consider the example given in Table 7.

Table 7

	Variable 1		Total
Variable 2	15		20
			50
Total	30	40	70

As you can see, any number less than 20 could have been chosen for the first cell. But once that number is fixed (at 15 in the example) there is no choice about what the empty cells should contain.

ACTIVITY 7

Show the calculation for the degrees of freedom for Table 3(a). (You will need to read Stats Piece 5 first.)

Let us now consider the final part of the jigsaw. Returning to the extract from the third reading, consider the χ^2 value for the retention interval of 98.42. You know, from Section 4.1, that *p* is the term for the *observed level of significance* which can be attached to the result. In our example the statement that *p* is less than .0001, expressed as $p < .0001$, means that if the null hypothesis that there is no association is not rejected, the probability that a chi-square value of at least that level occurring purely by chance is less than .0001, which, put another way, is less than one in 10,000. The researchers, not surprisingly, therefore concluded that the null hypothesis should be rejected.

The smaller *p* is, the more significant (in the statistical sense) the finding is and the less likely it is to have occurred by chance. It is always possible to draw a random sample from a population and pick an untypical one by chance, and so to produce findings for the sample which do not hold for the population. What the statistical test does is to assess the probability of having done so. Because the probability level in this particular instance is so small, it is highly unlikely that such a value for chi-square could have occurred by chance — there is less than one chance of it in 10,000. Therefore the hypothesis that the two variables are independent for this particular set of data — that there is no relationship between them — is rejected, and we describe the findings as *statistically significant*.

Putting all this another way, you can think of it as a kind of 'model-fitting'. What we are trying to do is to see how well our data correspond to the null hypothesis that the two variables are *not* associated in the population — that knowing the value of one does not help you to predict the value of the other.

STATS PIECE 5: CALCULATING DEGREES OF FREEDOM

Table 8 Degrees of freedom for a 3 × 4 table

		Variable 1				
		1	2	3	4	Total
Variable 2	1	20	25	45	60	150
	2	30	90	35	45	200
	3	50	25	80	35	190
Total		100	140	160	140	540

Look at Table 8 which shows a 3 × 4 table. The total for column one is 100. If we were choosing the numbers to go into the three cells in column one, we could freely choose any number less than 100 for the first cell, and again, any number less than (100 minus cell one) for the second cell. However, for the third cell, there would be no choice, as it would have to be whatever number was necessary to make the total for the column equal to 100 (see shaded cell). The same situation is true for columns two and three. The cells which make up column four are also the last cells of each of the three rows in the table, so they are all shaded because their values are determined by the other selections in the row.

The only cells free to vary are the unshaded ones, so we have six degrees of freedom for the table. The general rule is that the number of degrees of freedom for a row is the number of cells in the row, r, minus one: written as $r - 1$. Similarly the number of degrees of freedom for a column in a table is the number of cells in that column, c, minus one: $c - 1$. In other words, for a two-way table with r rows and c columns, the degree of freedom for that table would be:

$$df = (r - 1) \times (c - 1)$$

because while the contents of $(r - 1)$ and $(c - 1)$ rows and columns can vary, the final row and column on any table is then determined by what must be included to reach the specific marginal totals for that table. (You should note that the calculation for the degrees of freedom for a tri-variate table is a little more complicated.) If you only have one row or one column, then the calculation for the degrees of freedom would be $(c - 1)$ or $(r - 1)$ respectively.

STATS PIECE 6: CHI-SQUARE EXAMPLE

Table 9 Relationship between height and gender (fictional data)

Height	Observed values				Expected values					$\chi^2 = \Sigma \frac{(O-E)^2}{E}$		
	male	female	total	%	male	%	female	%	total	%	male	female	total
5'8"+	70	10	80	(40)	48	(40)	32	(40)	80	(40)	$\frac{(70-48)^2}{48} = 10.08$	$\frac{(10-32)^2}{32} = 15.12$	25.20
5'4"<5'8"	40	40	80	(40)	48	(40)	32	(40)	80	(40)	$\frac{(40-48)^2}{48} = 1.33$	$\frac{(40-32)^2}{32} = 2.00$	3.33
<5'4"	10	30	40	(20)	24	(20)	16	(20)	40	(20)	$\frac{(10-24)^2}{24} = 8.17$	$\frac{(30-16)^2}{16} = 12.25$	20.42
Total	120	80	200	(100)	120	(100)	80	(100)	200	(100)	19.58	29.37	48.95

$\chi^2 = 48.95$, with 2 df, $p < .001$

UNIT 19/20 ANALYSIS OF STRUCTURED DATA

> **Stats Piece 6 (continued)**
>
> Let the first block of Table 9 (observed values) be the figures for the height distribution for each gender that we actually obtain in the sample. The second block of the table is what we would expect the cell totals to be if gender and height were *not* associated with each other. If we could not predict height from gender information, or predict gender from information about height, then we would expect the height distribution for men and women separately to be no different from the height distribution for the sample as a whole. The contents of the two columns are therefore calculated from the percentage distribution of the 'total' sample column.
>
> We ask ourselves how different the two blocks are — how likely are we to get a random sample this different from the expected values by chance alone? To find out, we calculate χ^2 using the formula from Stats Piece 4 thus:
>
> > for each cell of the table we subtract the expected value from the observed one,
> >
> > square the result and
> >
> > divide by the expected value.
>
> Looking at the last column of the table (χ^2 total), you can see that if we add up all these figures, we get an overall χ^2 of 48.95.
>
> We now need to work out the degrees of freedom for this table using the method explained in Stats Piece 5. We see there are three rows and two columns in the observed values block of the table, so there are:
>
> $$df = (r - 1) \times (c - 1)$$
> $$= (3 - 1) \times (2 - 1) = 2 \times 1 = 2 \text{ degrees of freedom.}$$
>
> Looking up a χ^2 value of 48.95 in the χ^2 table in the Statistics Handbook (Section 5), with two degrees of freedom, we can see that the figure is 'significant at least to $p < .001$' — in other words, that we would get a value this different from the expected one less than once in 1,000 samples by chance alone. So the null hypothesis may be rejected.

ACTIVITY 8

Express in your own words the conclusions obtained from Tables 3(a), 3(b) and 4 as reported in the extract we have been looking at (reproduced below):

> By χ^2 the distribution of age groups is significantly different for all these variables: RI (χ^2 (10) = 98.42, $p < .0001$); grade (χ^2 (6) = 18.40, $p < .005$); and interest (χ^2 (4) = 10.90, $p < .02$).
>
> (Cohen et al., 1992b)

Examine the chi-square information about the variables and make notes on how it should be interpreted. Make sure you check the degrees of freedom and examine the p levels carefully.

It should be noted that the finding of an association between variables does not necessarily imply causality. For example, a study which examined parents' smoking habits and childrens' behaviour was reported in the national press as having found an association between the number of cigarettes smoked by mothers and the incidence of bad behaviour in the children. From this association, it would not be at all clear as to whether the bad behaviour drove the mothers to smoke more, or whether the sight of mothers smoking drove the children into rebellion. Or even, as we shall see later, whether the association was not a direct one at all, but the result for both mothers and children of an association with some other variable such as poverty or family stress. So in our case study, although we can see that age and retention interval, age and grade, and age and interest are each significantly associated, the chi-square measure does not indicate the actual strength or type of association between them, but merely the existence of an association.

You will have noticed in our consideration of the χ^2 information for the three different pairs of variables that it was the p values for each of the χ^2 values which were compared rather than the χ^2 values themselves. This is because the table dimensions and the sample sizes each so affect the calculated value of χ^2 that any comparison of the χ^2 measure itself for contingency tables of different sizes is meaningless. Because of this limitation, alternative measures of association which are based on χ^2 have been developed. These measures have in common the aim of achieving values which fall within a fixed range between 0 and 1 and also of minimizing the effects of table size and sample size. There are three key measures based on χ^2 which you are most likely to come across in research reports. The most frequently used measures for comparing the strength of the association between variables in different tables are the *phi coefficient,* often written as Φ (rhymes with why), the *coefficient of contingency C* and *Cramer's V.*

STATS PIECE 7: ALTERNATIVE MEASURES BASED ON χ^2

Phi coefficient

Φ is usually limited to 2 × 2 tables, mainly because of the fact that where either the row size or the column size is greater than two, Φ can fall outside the 0–1 range. It does, however, have the advantage of being relatively easy to calculate from χ^2:

$$\Phi = \sqrt{\frac{\chi^2}{N}}$$

where N is the number of cases in the data set.

Coefficient of contingency

The coefficient of contingency C:

$$C = \sqrt{\frac{\chi^2}{\chi^2 + N}}$$

has the slightly different problem of falling between 0 and something less than 1.

Cramer's V

Cramer's V is a variation of Φ:

$$V = \sqrt{\frac{\chi^2}{N(k - 1)}}$$

where k is either the number of rows or columns in the table, whichever is the smaller. V can reach the maximum level of 1.

Another use of chi-square which you will come across in research reports and journal articles is where it is used to test whether or not a sample distribution comes from a particular population. This is why chi-square is often called the *chi-square goodness of fit test.* Briefly, the chi-square test can be used to test the agreement or conformity between the frequencies which are actually achieved (or observed) in a sample for a particular attribute and the frequencies which would be expected from a theoretical distribution. For example, if a sample distribution was being tested against the population distribution. The expected frequencies are therefore known for the single attribute being examined. The null hypothesis H_0 would always be that the observed frequencies were the same as the population frequencies or the theoretical distribution from which the hypothesis suggests that it comes.

STATS PIECE 8: CHI-SQUARE AS A GOODNESS OF FIT TEST

The formula for chi-square as a goodness of fit test is exactly the same as when it is used to test for independence (see Stats Piece 4), i.e.

$$\chi^2 = \Sigma \frac{(O - E)^2}{E}.$$

For example, suppose the age profile for OU academic staff were as shown in Table 10.

Table 10 Goodness of fit of OU academic staff age profile with general population age profile (fictional data)

Age	General population %	Expected figure OU staff	Observed figure OU staff	O − E	$\frac{(O-E)^2}{E}$
<25	3.4	7	5	(2)[a]	4/7 = .57
25–29	8.0	16	14	(2)	4/16 = .25
30–34	11.0	22	20	(2)	4/22 = .18
35–39	17.9	36	42	6	36/36 = 1.00
40–44	25.4	51	58	7	49/51 = .96
45–49	17.0	34	45	11	121/34 = 3.56
50–54	8.9	18	10	(8)	64/18 = 3.56
55–59	5.7	11	4	(7)	49/11 = 4.45
60+	2.7	5	2	(3)	9/5 = 1.80
Total	100%	200	200		16.33

[a] Figures in parentheses indicate a negative number.

Therefore from Table 10, $\chi^2 = 16.33$.

Now H_0 is that $O = E$

    let $\alpha = .05$

and we have only one column of observed data, therefore we use

    $df = (r - 1)$

        $= (9 - 1) = 8$: the table has 8 degrees of freedom.

We reject H_0 if, for $\alpha = .05$ at 8 df, χ^2 is less than 16.33.

Now from Table 5 in the Statistics Handbook the χ^2 distribution tables for $\alpha = .05$ at 8 df, $\chi^2 = 15.51$ which is less than 16.33, therefore we reject H_0. Thus we would assert that the age distribution of the staff was not typical of the age distribution in the general population.

UNIT 19/20 ANALYSIS OF STRUCTURED DATA

ACTIVITY 9

You may need to do a goodness of fit χ^2 test (see Stats Piece 8) for a TMA, so let us try one out. (You will probably find it easiest to use the spreadsheet on FRAMEWORK, or even a hand calculator.) Below are sample percentages for gender in a hypothetical survey, and the figures for the population (Table 11). Fill in the rest of the table, and note briefly what your results mean.

Table 11 Goodness of fit between sample gender distribution and general population (fictional data)

Gender	Population %	Sample %	Sample frequency (observed)	Expected frequency	O – E	$\frac{(O - E)^2}{E}$
Male	49.0	52.4	786			
Female	51.0	47.6	714			
Total	100.0	100.0	1,500			$\chi^2 =$

4.3 z AND t TESTS

There are various tests which can be used to test different types of hypotheses. We have already looked at the chi-square test. In this section we will look briefly at two other commonly used tests, z and t tests, followed by a look at F tests in Section 4.4.

One of the simplest hypotheses which researchers would wish to examine would be the difference between two means. Consider, for instance, if researchers at the OU wished to compare the mean exam scores for students who had studied the recommended prerequisite course and for students who had not. The question they would need to address would be whether the difference between the two means could have arisen by chance, or was it a 'real', i.e. statistically significant, difference. One standard way of testing whether the difference between two means is significant or not is through the use of either the z test or Student's t-test. Remember that back in Section 3.3 we discussed how z-scores used standard deviations to transform measures into standard deviation units. A similar approach is used with the z test, which is so called because the difference between two means is converted into standard deviation units. You can see this more clearly if you read the formula for z in Stats Piece 9. This statistic has an approximately normal distribution which, you may recall, means that we can identify the likelihood of the null hypothesis, i.e. that the two means are equal. Unfortunately, if either of the two samples are smaller than 30, then the z statistic no longer approximates a normal distribution. Instead, the t statistic is used (this is often referred to as Student's t). In practice, with large samples, there are no differences between the z distribution and the t distribution. To use the t statistic however, you must take into account the degrees of freedom involved as its value is affected by the sample size. Both z and t tests are for use with variables measured on an interval or ratio scale. The test itself, whether z or t is used, allows the researcher to calculate the probability of a difference of that size occurring if the means were equal in the population from which the sample was drawn. The statistically significant difference would be one which resulted in a test value with an observed probability p of, say, < .05, in which case H_0 would be rejected.

> **STATS PIECE 9: HYPOTHESIS TESTING**
>
> To test the hypothesis that two population means for group 1 and group 2 are equal:
>
> $$z = \frac{\bar{x}_1 - \bar{x}_2}{\sqrt{\left(\frac{s_1^2}{n_1} + \frac{s_2^2}{n_2}\right)}}$$
>
> where
>
> $\bar{x}_1$ is the sample mean of group 1,
>
> $\bar{x}_2$ is the sample mean of group 2,
>
> s_1^2 is the sample variance of group 1,
>
> s_2^2 is the sample variance of group 2,
>
> n_1 is the sample size of group 1,
>
> n_2 is the sample size of group 2,
>
> and where n_1 and n_2 are greater than about 30. If n_1 and n_2 are less than about 30 then the following formula would be used:
>
> $$t = \frac{\bar{x}_1 - \bar{x}_2}{\sqrt{\left(\frac{(n_1 - 1)s_1^2 + (n_2 - 1)s_2^2}{n_1 + n_2 - 2}\right)\left(\frac{n_1 + n_2}{n_1 n_2}\right)}}$$
>
> with $(n_1 + n_2 - 2)$ df.
>
> Note that the z statistic is interpreted through the use of z tables, and the t statistic through t tables for the appropriate degrees of freedom. Both sets of tables are included in your Statistics Handbook.

We have been discussing z and t tests for *any* differences between pairs of means, whether they represented increases or decreases. These are termed *two-tailed* tests. However, it should be noted that if we were only interested in one of the directions, such as, say, whether grades were higher for the middle-aged than for the young, then a *one-tailed* test might be used. This merely means that the significance level α would need to be divided by 2 (making it even less likely that differences between sample means occur by chance), so a test value yielding a two-tailed p of .05 would give a one-tailed p of .025 (remember the shaded areas in Figures 6 and 7).

Let us look briefly at an example for interpreting t and z. The stages the researchers would have to go through in order to test their hypothesis would include:

1. Setting up the null hypothesis.
2. Deciding on the most appropriate test to assess that hypothesis.
3. Calculating the result of the test.
4. Setting the probability level α.
5. Comparing the probability of obtaining the test result against the α level.
6. Deciding whether to accept or reject the null hypothesis.

Suppose that researchers were investigating gender differences in exam results. In a small study of marks achieved by students for a particular exam, they reported that the analysis of the marks achieved by the 16 males and 16 females involved in the study were:

for 16 women: mean marks = 17.5, standard deviation = 3,

for 16 men: mean marks = 15.0, standard deviation = 4.

1 The null hypothesis H_0 is that the mean for women = mean for men.

2 Because n_1 and n_2 (sample sizes) are each less than 30, the researchers use Student's *t*-test to test their hypothesis. We are also interested in differences in *either* direction so we will be using a two-tailed *t* test.

3 The result for the *t* test on the data using the formula in Stats Piece 9 is $t = 2$. The degrees of freedom are:

$$n_1 + n_2 - 2 = 16 + 16 - 2 = 30 \; df.$$

4 We decide that the probability level α should be set at 5 per cent, i.e. $\alpha = .05$.

5 Reading the *t* table in the Statistics Handbook (Table 3) we find that at the 30 *df* level the probability of *t* being greater than 1.697 = .10, and the probability of *t* being greater than 2.042 = .05. Since we have calculated that $t = 2$, the probability of it occurring by chance is less than .10 (10 per cent) but greater than .05 (5 per cent).

6 Since we had previously decided to set α at 5 per cent, and we know that the probability of $t = 2$ is greater than 5 per cent, then the difference is *not* significant and we do not reject the null hypothesis (though the researchers would undoubtedly comment on the narrow margin of rejection and the fact that the samples were so small).

ACTIVITY 10

In the example above the researchers were investigating whether there were *any* differences between exam results achieved by men and women. Suppose, however, that they wanted to investigate whether women achieved higher exam results than men.

1 What sort of test would be needed?

2 What would be the effect on how *p* is interpreted?

ACTIVITY 11

If you found this section difficult, try working through the NUMERACY computer-assisted learning disk, Topic 3.

4.4 ANALYSIS OF VARIANCE

While *z* and *t* tests are fine for examining two means at a time, there can be problems where differences between a number of sample means are being investigated. If we go back to the contingency tables we were examining earlier (Tables 3a and 3b), you can see that they each contain a 'mean' column. Readers are given the mean grades for each age grouping (Table 3a) and the mean level of interest for each age grouping (Table 3b). A brief scan of the tables suggests that there appears to be a relationship with age for both grade and interest. The question is whether the difference between, say, the mean grade of 2.43 achieved by former students classified as 'young' and the mean grade of 2.92 achieved by former students classified as 'elderly' is a 'real' difference in the statistical sense, or whether it could have arisen by chance.

The problem here is that testing several mean differences one by one invites Type 1 error. If our α is set at .05, for example, all this says is that we should not get a falsely significant result more often than one time in 20; so if we do 20 tests, it is statistically likely that at least one of them will have given a falsely significant result. The usual solution to this situation is the one described in the third reading. The researchers wish to investigate significant differences between a number of sample means. The procedure Cohen *et al.* used was *one-way analysis of variance*.

The two pieces of information needed to describe a distribution, namely a measure of the central tendency such as the mean and a measure of the spread such as the standard deviation or variance, play a key role when it comes to drawing conclusions about a population from the results obtained through hypothesis testing. We can use information about the variance of each of the samples when examining the means of several different populations for any significant differences. The total variance of the data in all the samples is split into two parts: that due to the variance *between* the samples and that due to the variance *within* the samples. This is in effect the principle underlying analysis of variance. The ratio of these two parts of the total variance is known as F. If the calculated value of F is found to be significant, then it is assumed that the differences between the means are also significant.

In Table 12 the mean of the test scores achieved by respondents in each of the three age groups are given for each of the eight tests used. The question being investigated is whether the differences identified in the mean test scores between the people in each age group are attributable to chance, or whether they represent real differences between the groups. In other words, is age a significant factor in students' test performance? If it is, then the mean scores for different age groups will not be equal. The null hypothesis H_0, in other words, is that the populations from which the samples have been drawn all have equal means, i.e. that any differences there are between the sample mean scores for each age group are likely to have arisen by chance. The test for this hypothesis is the F test.

Table 12 Mean percentage correct response, by age

Test	Young	Middle	Elderly	Chance[a]	F [b]
Name recognition	71	66	66	50	6.12
Concept recognition	72	69	68	50	5.32
Fact verification general	67	65	65	50	NS
Fact verification specific	71	65	64	50	7.19
Grouping	43	36	34	17	4.70
Cued recall names	37	29	27	0	NS
Cued recall concepts	42	32	24	0	11.73
Experimental design	76	77	74	50	NS

[a] The 'chance' column indicates the score achievable by picking answers at random.
[b] All F values are significant at $p < .001$.
(Source: Cohen et al., 1992b, Table 2)

If the null hypothesis of equal means is not rejected, then the expected ratio of the two parts of the total variance will be $F = 1$. In Table 12 three F values are identified as 'NS', i.e. 'not significant'. In other words, differences in sample means do not suggest there are differences between age groups in the larger population for those particular tests. The calculated values for F for the other listed test-means range from 4.70 to 11.73. The given p level is < 0.001, this means that the probability of obtaining just by chance an F value at least as large as the ones calculated is less than 0.001, i.e. less than one in 1,000. In other words, the F values suggest strongly that there are real differences between the means of the different age groups. The question then arises for each of the tests as to which of the means of the three age groups do differ significantly from each other.

STATS PIECE 10: ONE WAY ANALYSIS OF VARIANCE

When testing the means of different groups the variance s^2 will comprise two parts:

1. the variation of the means between groups, the measure of which is the *between-groups sum of squares*, and
2. the variability of the measures within each group, the measure of which is the *within-groups sum of squares* (also sometimes called the error sum of squares).

The hypothesis H_0 being tested is that the means of all the groups are equal, i.e. that any differences between means are not significant. The test used for this is the F test:

$$F = \frac{\text{between-groups mean square}}{\text{within-groups mean square}}$$

where mean squares are in effect the means of the sum of squares. They are calculated by dividing each sum of squares by the appropriate number of degrees of freedom. So the between-groups degrees of freedom is $k - 1$ where k is the number of groups; and the within-groups degrees of freedom is $n - k$ where n is the number of cases in the total sample.

The summary of the sequence of calculations for F can perhaps be seen most clearly with the use of the analysis of variance (ANOVA) table as follows (Table 13).

Table 13 One-way ANOVA table

Source	df	Sum of squares (SS)	Mean squares (MS)	F ratio
Between groups (explained variation)	$k - 1$	SS (between groups) $= \sum_{i=1}^{k} n_i(\bar{x}_i - \bar{x})^2$	$\dfrac{\text{SS (between groups)}}{k - 1}$	$\dfrac{\text{MS (between groups)}}{\text{MS (within groups)}}$
Within groups (residual variation)	$n - k$	SS (within groups) $= \sum_{i=1}^{k} (n_i - 1)s_i^2$ where s_i^2 is the variance of group i about its mean	$\dfrac{\text{SS (within groups)}}{n - k}$	
Total	$n - 1$	SS (total)		

It is after having found significant values of F that pairs of means should be tested. At this point, while we know there are significant differences somewhere between the group means, we do not know which of the groups are the ones which differ significantly from each other. The researchers report in the third reading that they tested individual pairs of scores using a procedure called Fisher's LSD test, one of a number of techniques devised for this purpose. Multiple comparison tests such as this have been devised in such a way as to minimize the chance of either Type 1 or Type 2 errors. It is clearly good practice to carry out a preliminary analysis of variance in this way so that the significant F ratios can be identified through the analysis of all the groups, before comparing individual pairs of means. By doing so we do just a single test to find out whether there is sufficient variance between groups to explain, before trying to locate where it lies.

The next step in analysis reported in Cohen *et al.* (1992b) is the *two-way analysis of variance*. This is used for data which is grouped using two variables rather than just the one (age) used for the one-way analysis of variance (ANOVA). The two variables used in the reading are age and retention interval.

Again, the total variance is being split into its component parts. However, this time, because the effects of two independent variables are being investigated, the possibility of each of them affecting the other as well as there being a possible association between each of the independent variables and the dependent variable must be taken into account. In the particular example in the third reading, we already know that there is some interaction between these two variables as the correlation between them has already been shown to be significant (we will be discussing correlation in the next section). If we carried out the same procedure as for one-way analysis of variance, and a significant difference was found, we would have no way of knowing whether this was due to differences between the age groups, the retention intervals, or to both of them. This is called a *confounding* effect. In order to take account of the joint effects of the two independent variables acting together, an additional variance component is included in the formula. This means that F ratios then have to be calculated for the interaction as well as for separate contributions which each of the two independent variables may make (known as *main effects*).

Suppose, for example, that we were interested in examining the effects of gender and height on promotion. There would be three sets of hypotheses which could be tested using a two-way design:

H_{01}: gender is not a factor in promotion,

H_{02}: height is not a factor in promotion, and

H_{03}: the interaction between height and gender is not a factor in promotion.

There will be a number of possible degrees of freedom depending on which hypothesis is being tested. In addition, because we are dealing with the ratio of two parts of the total variance when we use the F test, we will be handling two sets of degrees of freedom when we come to interpret the F statistic: the set arising from the factor whose effect is being tested (V_1) and the set arising from the unexplained variation (V_2). If you look in your Statistics Handbook at Table 6(b), you will see how the values of F at $p < .01$ or at $p < .05$ (Table 6a) are determined by the degrees of freedom V_1 and V_2. For example, suppose we have a computed F statistic of $F = 2.59$. If we have set $\alpha = 0.05$, and we know our degrees of freedom are $V_1 = 3$ and $V_2 = 28$, then we can read from the table that $F(3,28)$ for $\alpha = 0.05$ is 2.95. This is sometimes written in research journals as $F_{.05,3,28} = 2.95$. Comparing the two figures we can see that our computed $F = 2.59 < 2.95$, so we would not reject our H_0.

ACTIVITY 12

Read the following extract from the third reading.

> Main effects of RI were significant for name recognition (F (5,355) = 9.07, $p < .001$); concept recognition (F (5,355) = 18.57, $p < .001$); fact verification specific (F (5,355) = 2.41, $p < .05$); grouping (F (5,355) = 6.30, $p < .001$); cued recall of names (F (5,355) = 3.95, $p < .001$); and for cued recall of concepts (F (5,355) = 6.95, $p < .001$).
>
> (Cohen et al., 1992b)

Explain what this extract is saying.

Analysis of variance can be used with even more independent variables. The techniques are more complex and varied but the principles are the same. The strength of ANOVA is that it relies on the additive properties of sample variances. However, three criteria must be met to check the appropriateness of analysis of variance for specific data sets:

1   All observations should be independent of each other — that is, no individual should appear twice in the data set.

2   The populations from which the samples are drawn should be normally distributed.

3   The groups should have the same within-groups variance (because the estimate of the population within-groups variance will be biased if the variances differ widely).

The great strength of this technique is that it can deal with all types of data — nominal, ordinal, interval and ratio. However, the *dependent* variable must be interval level while the independent variables are treated as nominal variables. Its great weakness is that in its simplest form it requires all the groups to be the same size. This is not a problem in experimental research, where equal-sized groups can generally be arranged, but in survey analysis it is rarely the case that groups to be compared are of equal size. There are forms of analysis of variance which can cope with this, but for the most part their use is valid only under very restricted circumstances, so analysis of variance as a technique is not much used in survey analysis. However, the *principles* underlying analysis of variance also underlie several other important analysis techniques, and understanding them is therefore as important for survey researchers as for experimenters.

5   CORRELATION AND REGRESSION

5.1   CORRELATION COEFFICIENTS

As you saw earlier, there are a number of measures of association based on chi-square. All assume only that the variables are nominal. However, as you may have noted in Activity 2, the variables in Tables 3(a), 3(b) and 4 are not nominal. Thus age as presented in the tables is an ordinal variable, as is the retention interval, while grade is an ordinal or possibly interval variable and interest an ordinal variable. You will sometimes see examples of researchers using χ^2 with ordinal and other types of data. This is perfectly valid statistically, but information about the data is being lost where this occurs because chi-square only identifies the existence of an association and not its type or strength. The additional information which ordinal, interval and ratio variables hold can be used to give us a better idea of the strength and type of association between them. Of particular importance here is the form of association known as *correlation*. A correlation is simply the association between two variables. Look at Figure 8 which gives a simple example of a small data set shown as a scattergram which plots the data and which shows visually the association between two variables age and height.

If a high value on one variable is associated with a high value on another (for example with height and age in children), they are said to be *positively* correlated. If a high value on one variable is associated with a lower value on the other, then they are said to be *negatively* correlated (for example age and energy!).

In Cohen *et al.* (1992b) the discussion of the data examines the chi-square results, then moves on to look in more detail at the association between age and retention interval. The index or the statistic which is used to indicate the *strength* of the association between these two variables is the *correlation coefficient r*. Just as the

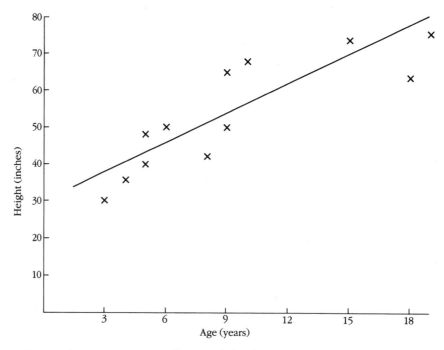

Figure 8 *A scattergram (fictional data)*

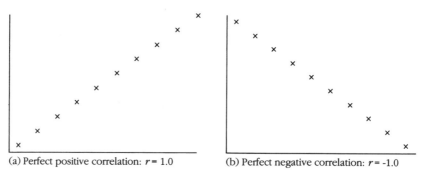

(a) Perfect positive correlation: $r = 1.0$ (b) Perfect negative correlation: $r = -1.0$

Figure 9 *Perfect correlations*

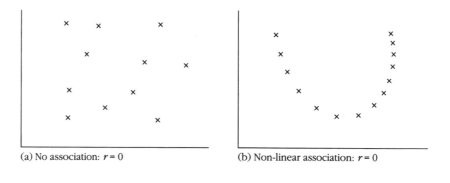

(a) No association: $r = 0$ (b) Non-linear association: $r = 0$

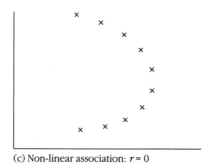

(c) Non-linear association: $r = 0$

Figure 10 *Associations where* $r = 0$

mean and variance give a useful summary description of one distribution, the correlation coefficient gives a useful summary description of the association between any two distributions. Pearson's product moment correlation coefficient r is the most commonly used correlation coefficient used for interval data. It can take values from +1 to −1, by which means it indicates how close to linearity the association is. 'Linear' is just the statistical term for a straight line, so a linear correlation means that the measures for the pair of variables being investigated, together form a straight line (see Figure 9).

The fact that Pearson's r measures only linear correlations is an important feature of this particular index. Figure 10 gives three *scattergrams* which each show a set of measures for pairs of variables for individual respondents. These scattergrams show examples of different types of associations which can be found between pairs of variables. As you can see, a correlation of $r = 0$ in Figure 10(a) reflects the fact that there is no linear association between the two variables. However, as Figures 10(b) and (c) also show, there could well be a non-linear association. That is, scores on one variable may be predictable from scores on another (though perhaps not uniquely), but because there is no simple one-to-one linear relationship between scores, the correlation coefficient would still be zero.

STATS PIECE 11: PEARSON'S CORRELATION COEFFICIENT

Pearson's product moment correlation coefficient is defined as:

$$r = \frac{\Sigma(x_i - \bar{x})(y_i - \bar{y})}{(n - 1)s_X s_Y}$$

where

Σx_i = sum over all the n measurements of variable X, and

Σy_i = sum over all the n measurements of variable Y,

for a data set of n values with standard deviation of s_X for X and s_Y for Y.

So

$$r = \frac{\text{sum of squares for } XY}{(\sqrt{\text{sum of squares for } X})(\sqrt{\text{sum of squares for } Y})}.$$

ACTIVITY 13

If you found these ideas difficult, work through Topic 4 on the NUMERACY disk.

There are a variety of forms of correlation coefficients which have been developed for different types of variables. For interval or ratio data such as test scores, Pearson's r is the most widely used. For ranked ordinal or non-normal interval data the most frequently used measure is Spearman's rank order correlation coefficient r_s.

So how is r interpreted? A value of 1 would indicate a perfect association. This would be a highly unlikely result and would be the cause for concern and questioning if it occurred. Far more likely are correlations around the 0.1, 0.2 level which would be taken to indicate no association. A correlation of $r = 0.8$ would indicate a strong association. However if, for example, it was reported that two variables had an r of .3, then the interpretation would be less clear and would depend on whether or not r was found to be statistically significant. Like all other statistics, if the aim of getting the correlation coefficient in a sample is to test hypotheses about an unknown population correlation coefficient ρ (rho, pronounced roe), then the correlation coefficient r must be tested for statistical significance. The hypothesis, H_0, being tested would be that in the population the correlation coefficient is zero; in other words that there was no correlation between the two variables. Checking the statistical significance of r is simply a matter of looking up the value of r for the appropriate number of degrees of freedom ($n - 2$) in the critical values table. Section 4 in your Statistics Handbook explains in detail how you do this. Alternatively, the significance of r may be calculated by using t, as shown in Stats Piece 12.

Thus for any value of the correlation coefficient calculated from a sample, the likelihood that there is a positive linear correlation can be tested using the t test in the usual way with $df = n - 2$ (the formula is given in Stats Piece 12).

STATS PIECE 12: USING t TO TEST THE SIGNIFICANCE OF PEARSON'S r

For any given r, when n is the number of measurements in the sample,

$$t = r \sqrt{\left(\frac{n - 2}{1 - r^2}\right)}$$

with $n - 2$ degrees of freedom.

Let us look at a brief example.

Our null hypothesis H_0 will be that there is no linear relationship between the two variables in the population from which the sample is drawn. This means we are looking at a two-tailed test for t where H_0: $\rho = 0$ (where ρ is the population correlation coefficient).

Say $r = 0.3$ and $n = 30$, then

$$df = n - 2 = 30 - 2 = 28$$

$$t = 0.3 \sqrt{\left(\frac{30 - 2}{1 - (0.3)^2}\right)}$$

$$= 0.3 \sqrt{\left(\frac{28}{0.91}\right)}$$

$$= 0.3 \sqrt{30.77} = 0.3 \times 5.55 = 1.66.$$

Looking up t in the Statistics Handbook we find that for a two-tailed test with 28 df, $p < .2$ for $t = 1.66$. This means that the probability of this occurring by chance is less than 20 per cent (.2). The correlation is therefore not significant and we do not reject the null hypothesis.

We do not reject H_0 and conclude that there is no linear relationship between the two variables being examined.

5.2 SIMPLE LINEAR REGRESSION

We have already seen that if it is possible to construct a straight line through data points on a scattergram, we can use the information it gives us about the relationship between the two variables in order to estimate or predict the behaviour of one variable from the other. In Figure 8 a rough line was drawn 'by eye' to indicate the best prediction of height from age. Using the computational power of a computer it is possible to fit a prediction line to the data much more rigorously and precisely.

The convention is that the dependent variable is usually shown on the vertical (or Y axis), and the independent (or explanatory) variable is shown on the X axis. Consider the data from the research reported in the readings. We might expect that at a given time those people who have only been away from the course for a relatively short time — that is, those with only a short retention interval — would have more accurate recall of aspects of the course than those who finished the course some years earlier. If we plotted the test results data on the Y axis, and the retention interval on the X axis, as a scattergram, we might expect to see a positive correlation in the form of a linear association. However, it is equally clear that any attempt to draw a straight line through the data points on the scattergram would leave many of the points near rather than actually on the line. It is therefore necessary to make sure that a line is drawn which minimizes the distances of the data points from the line, by drawing the *line of best fit*. Figure 11 illustrates three such lines — a perfect fit, a good fit and a poor fit to the data set (because the data points are *not* randomly scattered about the line so the average distance of the data points from the line will not be zero as they would be with a good fit). Even though there is a fair degree of variability with the good fit, the average distance of the data points from the line *do* add up to zero. In other words, the line is positioned in such a way as to achieve the least variation possible among the residuals. This line is called the *linear regression line*.

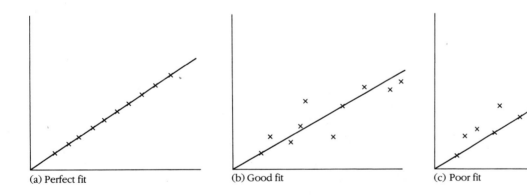

(a) Perfect fit (b) Good fit (c) Poor fit

Figure 11 *Lines of best fit*

STATS PIECE 13: REGRESSION LINES

The equation for fitting a regression line is

$$\hat{Y} = a + bX$$

where

$\hat{Y}$ is the measure or score which we want to predict,

a is the point at which the regression line cuts the Y axis, and

b is the slope or the gradient of the line, i.e. the number of units of Y the line goes up for each unit of X and is called the *regression coefficient*.

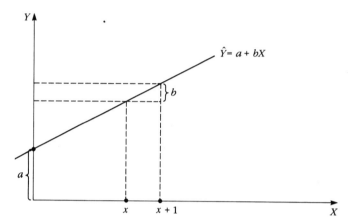

Figure 12 *Linear regression line and the regression coefficient*

A regression line predicts Y-values from X-values.

For example, a regression line for length of babies (in inches) by age (in days) might be specified by

$$\hat{Y} = 15 + 0.5X$$

where $\hat{Y}$ is length of the baby and X is the age of the baby.

This would be interpreted as saying that babies are 15 inches long on average at birth (when $X = 0$ and a, the intercept, is 15 inches) and grow by (say) half an inch each day (i.e. b, the regression coefficient, is 0.5 inches).

However, as you saw in Figure 11(c), the fit of a regression line to any data is very unlikely to be perfect. This means that the predicted measure will usually be different from the actual measure at any particular point. This variability in the actual data which is 'unexplained' by the line can be expressed as:

$$\Sigma(\hat{Y} - Y)$$

where

$\hat{Y}$ is the predicted measure (e.g. predicted length at a given age), and

Y is the actual measure (e.g. actual length at a given age).

The full regression equation should be written as:

$Y = \hat{Y}$ + residual (as shown in Figure 13)

substituting for $\hat{Y}$ this would give

$= a + bX$ + residual.

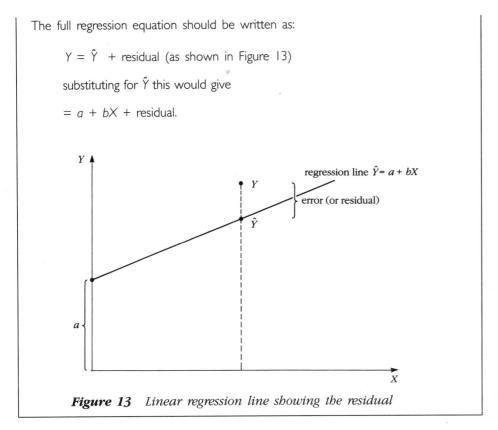

Figure 13 *Linear regression line showing the residual*

Having computed the regression line, we now need a measure of how *good* a fit it is. That is how much residual variance is left after we subtract the variance explained by the regression. This measure, in fact, is provided by r, the correlation coefficient. As we saw in Section 5.1, the correlation coefficient expresses the extent to which the data points cluster about the regression line (see Figure 14).

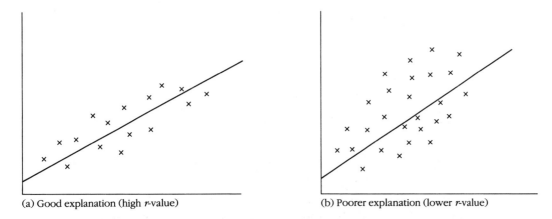

(a) Good explanation (high r-value) (b) Poorer explanation (lower r-value)

Figure 14 *Correlation as a measure of variance explained*

The nearer the data points are to the line, the higher the correlation. So when regression analysis is used, a correlation coefficient is cited as an estimate of how much of the variance is explained by the analysis. Squaring the correlation coefficient gives us the proportion of the variance explained in the dependent variable; so for example, a correlation of $r = 0.7$ explains 0.49 of the variance (49 per cent). The square of the correlation coefficient is known as the *coefficient of determination* and is often written as r^2 for the simple linear model.

Basically, regression analysis explains the sources of variance of the dependent variable Y. If we say that the total variance of Y is 1, then the proportion of the variance *not* accounted for by the coefficient of determination will be $1 - r^2$. The proportion of the variance which is not accounted for represents the residual variance. It is this variance which researchers seek to minimize when they construct a linear regression line.

6 MULTIVARIATE ANALYSES

The last task of this unit is to consider the extension of these statistics to situations where we need to take account of more than one independent variable — in other words where researchers need to use multivariate analyses. The normal research question in social research usually needs a multivariate approach; few research problems are so neatly circumscribed that we can identify and test a single cause or influence. Many research papers look at a number of possible influences on the dependent variable to be explained. Some just examine these influences one at a time, to show whether each bears a significant relationship to the dependent variable, but this does not tell the reader a great deal. We really need to know:

1. which of the influences are strong and which are weak,

2. to what extent the different independent variables are *independent* influences (or, conversely, how much their influence overlaps), and

3. whether there are *interaction effects* (whether the influence of two or more variables together is different from what would be predicted of any one solely by itself).

Another reason why we might want to involve more than one potential independent variable in our analysis is that experiments are relatively rare in social and educational research. In a true experiment it is possible to select groups which are arguably identical on everything except the 'treatment' variable — by matching or by random allocation. In 'real world' research we are more often comparing groups which differ in a number of respects as well as the one which is of interest to us. Lacking the *design* controls of experimental studies, we therefore need multivariate analysis techniques for the *statistical* control of these 'unwanted' differences. In other words, we need to show:

1. whether the effects of extraneous variables are larger than those of the influence(s) we are studying,

2. whether they are *confounded* with them (that is, highly correlated with them), and

3. whether they *interact* with them.

There are broadly two 'families' of multivariate techniques — the analysis of variance family and the regression family. You were introduced to the ideas behind each of these 'families', and to the relationship between them, in previous sections of the unit. Each 'family' is illustrated below by discussing one or two members in some detail and then covering more briefly other variants which you might well encounter in research papers. The two 'families' aim to perform very similar tasks — and indeed are closely related mathematically, for the most part — but they have different strengths and weaknesses. Both aim to establish which of the variables have the strongest effects, and generally to estimate the proportion of the variance in the dependent variable which is 'explained' by each independent variable. Regression techniques concentrate on linear relationships and are weaker at exploring interaction effects. Analysis of variance techniques are strong for exploring interaction effects but do not provide such precise predictions of linear causal factors. In this section of the unit we look briefly at a range of the most common multivariate techniques.

6.1 TABULAR TECHNIQUES

At the risk of seeming deliberately paradoxical, we might count the use of tabular analysis and χ^2 as a member of the analysis of variance family — the simplest member, but showing a family resemblance to its more grown-up siblings. Thinking back to Section 4.2 you may recall how, like analysis of variance, χ^2 is a 'model-fitting' technique; it tests the null hypothesis that the observed pattern in a table could plausibly be written off as a chance sample from a population in which the pattern would not be observed. In other words, χ^2 tests the hypothesis of random distribution between columns and rows of tables in the same way that analysis of variance tests the null hypothesis of random distribution between groups.

Chi-square enables you to say that an observed association is significant — that the observed association has a low probability of occurring by chance alone. Thus the first stage in a multivariate tabular analysis would be to tabulate each independent variable separately against the dependent variable and compute χ^2 for each table. This would enable you, perhaps, to discard some variables as not showing a significant relationship with the dependent variable. If all your tables have the same degrees of freedom you can also compute Φ for 2×2 tables, or some other coefficient association for tables of a different size, and compare these. This will tell you which of the independent variables has the *strongest* effect (the largest χ^2). The Φ coefficient (which was introduced in Section 4.2) can be used to make a rough estimate of how much variance each explains. As with r^2, Φ^2 gives an estimate of the proportion of variance explained, but gives a much rougher estimate than r would provide. You can take tabular analysis further, and use it to explore for interaction effects and confounded extraneous variables, by partitioning your tables by a third variable.

The following is an extended example, prepared by Roger Sapsford based on an analysis presented in Unit 16, the 'pay-off' of educational qualifications in terms of wages earned. The data came from the 1980–4 responses to the Open University's People in Society survey. (Note that the χ^2 values reproduced here were calculated from the original raw numbers, of course, not the percentages shown in the tables.)

Extended example

Table 14, in its first block, looks at the relationship of educational qualifications to current income. There is a significant and reasonably strong relationship ($\Phi = 0.32$, and Φ tends to underestimate association). Looking at the 'total' block of the table, about two-thirds of people with few or no qualifications have 'low' incomes (defined as 'below the median' for the total sample), and about two-thirds of people with higher qualifications have 'high' incomes. In the other two blocks of the table we look separately at males and females — we 'control for gender' — and see that the relationship holds good for both. Women more often have *low* incomes than men — substantially more women than men appear in the first column of their respective blocks — but within that constraint the relationship holds. So far, therefore, we have a two-factor explanation of wage levels: women earn less than men, but for both education brings rewards. (If the χ^2 in the male and female blocks of the table had both been non-significant, we should have concluded that gender, not educational level, was the determining factor. If they had come out as of very different sizes, we should have concluded that there was an interaction effect at work, the size of the relationship being effected by the value on the 'gender' variable.)

Table 14 The 'pay-off' of education: wages and educational qualifications, in total and by gender

	Total		Males		Females	
Education	low wages	high wages	low wages	high wages	low wages	high wages
O level or less	% 62.9	37.1	% 44.2	55.8	% 82.3	17.7
More than O level	% 31.2	68.8	% 15.9	84.1	% 46.8	53.2
	$n = 4{,}632$		$n = 2{,}307$		$n = 2{,}325$	
	$\chi^2 = 472.02$, $df = 1$, $p < .0001$		$\chi^2 = 220.81$, $df = 1$, $p < .0001$		$\chi^2 = 324.70$, $df = 1$, $p < .0001$	
	$\Phi = 0.32$		$\Phi = 0.31$		$\Phi = 0.37$	

Table 15 splits each half of the sample by whether or not they are in full-time work. For men, as we can see, this makes a crucial difference; there are relatively few men not in full-time work, and among them there is no statistically significant association of education with wages. For women there are also fairly marked differences, but even in the 'not' category the sample is large enough that a relatively low association comes out as statistically significant. Even among women with part-time jobs, therefore, education has some tendency to be associated with higher income. There is clearly an interaction between educational level and being in full- or part-time work, however, and the latter is a confounded variable which is distorting the analysis. We can correct this by looking only at *full-time* workers (Table 16).

Table 15 Wages and educational level by gender and job status

	Males full time		Males not full time		Females full time		Females not full time	
Education	low wages	high wages	low wages	high wages	low wages	high wages	low wages	high wages
O level or less	% 35.3	64.7	% 86.4	13.6	% 66.2	33.8	% 94.0	6.0
More than O level	% 11.4	88.6	% 76.5	23.5	% 27.4	72.6	% 85.3	14.7
	$n = 2{,}028$		$n = 279$		$n = 1{,}223$		$n = 1{,}102$	
	$\chi^2 = 164.21$, $df = 1$, $p < .0001$		$\chi^2 = 3.34$, $df = 1$, NS		$\chi^2 = 182.37$, $df = 1$, $p < .0001$		$\chi^2 = 21.60$, $df = 1$, $p < .0001$	
	$\Phi = 0.28$		$\Phi = 0.11$		$\Phi = 0.39$		$\Phi = 0.14$	

Table 16 Wages and educational level by gender, for full-time workers

Education	Total		Males		Females	
	low wages	high wages	low wages	high wages	low wages	high wages
O level or less	% 46.9	53.1	% 35.3	64.7	% 66.2	33.8
More than O level	% 17.5	82.5	% 11.4	88.6	% 27.4	72.6
	$n = 3{,}251$		$n = 2{,}028$		$n = 1{,}223$	
	$\chi^2 = 461.55$, $df = 1$, $p < .0001$		$\chi^2 = 164.21$, $df = 1$, $p < .0001$		$\chi^2 = 182.37$, $df = 1$, $p < .0001$	
	$\Phi = 0.38$		$\Phi = 0.28$		$\Phi = 0.39$	

As in Table 14 we find a significant and reasonably strong relationship for both sexes, though again women tend overall to earn less than men; the lower apparent level of women's wages was not just due to the larger proportion of them working part-time or not at all. We may also note an interaction effect, however: the association is substantially higher for women than for men. This is in line with other research on women's work suggesting that the level of women's jobs is better predicted by initial qualifications than men's because men receive more 'promotion on the job'.

Finally, in Table 17 we explore the effects of a fourth variable, marital status. It might be hypothesized that because married women often take jobs at below their 'true' level, the relationship would break down for married women. In fact this hypothesis appears disproved. The relationship is significant in all four blocks of the table, but lowest for *unmarried men*. One further variable which might be worth exploring here is age: as women on the whole marry younger than men, the unmarried females in the table may be more homogeneous with respect to age than the unmarried men, and as age affects earnings (though possibly more for men than women), this may be an alternative explanation for the results in Table 17.

Table 17 Wages and educational level by gender (full-time workers) and marital statistics

Education	Males married		Males not married		Females married		Females not married	
	low wages	high wages	low wages	high wages	low wages	high wages	low wages	high wages
O level or less	% 27.4	72.6	% 49.0	51.0	% 58.8	41.2	% 74.4	25.6
More than O level	% 5.1	94.9	% 25.8	74.2	% 22.7	77.3	% 31.3	68.8
	$n = 1{,}356$		$n = 672$		$n = 593$		$n = 630$	
	$\chi^2 = 129.72$, $df = 1$, $p < .0001$		$\chi^2 = 37.40$, $df = 1$, $p < .0001$		$\chi^2 = 78.6$, $df = 1$, $p < .0001$		$\chi^2 = 112.43$, $df = 1$, $p < .0001$	
	$\Phi = 0.31$		$\Phi = 0.24$		$\Phi = 0.36$		$\Phi = 0.42$	

From this extended example then, you can see how tabular analysis, conceptually the simplest of the multivariate analyses, can deliver quite a lot of what we need. It can tell us which variables relate significantly to the criterion (the dependent variable), roughly how strong the relationship between variables is, which relationships are stronger than others, and even whether there are interaction effects. The estimate of strength of relationship is only a rough one, however, and tabular analysis cannot estimate at all the proportion of variance explained by interaction effects. For this we need more sensitive and precise techniques.

6.2 MORE ON ANALYSIS OF VARIANCE

The best known of such techniques is *analysis of variance* itself. As we saw in Section 4.4, one-way analysis of variance can be extended into two-way analysis of variance, and it can be extended again to include multiple dependent variables. With one-way ANOVA, the hypothesis tested is that for one particular variable the means of all the groups are equal: i.e. that the populations from which the groups are drawn have equal means. For example, that different age groups scored equally well on a factual recall test. With two-way ANOVA, we saw earlier how two factors are explored, by looking at an example of the effects of both height and gender on promotion. As we saw, the major difference between one-way and two-way analyses was that we now had to consider not just the effects of each individual factor, but also the possible *interaction* effects. Look at the following extract from the third reading. You will already be familiar with part of this extract as you were asked to analyse a section of it in Activity 12.

> Two-way analyses of variance were also performed for each test with age and RI as between-subjects factors. Age was grouped into young, middle-aged and elderly, and RI was grouped into two-year intervals. Main effects of RI were significant for name recognition ($F(5,355) = 9.07$, $p < .001$); concept recognition ($F(5,355) = 18.57$, $p < .001$); fact verification specific ($F(5,355) = 2.41$, $p < .05$); grouping ($F(5,355) = 6.30$, $p < .001$); cued recall of names ($F(5,355) = 3.95$, $p < .001$); and for cued recall of concepts ($F(5,355) = 6.95$, $p < .001$). The effects of RI were not significant in the test of fact verification general nor in the test of experimental design. The main effect of age was significant only in two of the tests, fact verification specific ($F(2,355) = 3.05$, $p < .05$) and, marginally, in cued recall of concepts ($F(2,355) = 2.41$, $p < .09$). The interaction of age × RI did not approach significance in any of the tests. It is clear that the age differences which emerged from the one-way analyses of variance are much less evident when RI is included as a factor and this is due to the fact that, as shown in Table 1a, age and RI are highly correlated.
>
> (Cohen *et al.*, 1992b)

Here you will see that a series of eight two-way analyses of variance were carried out — one for each of the individual tests. In each computation, the test score was the dependent variable, with age and the retention interval as the two independent variables. Remember that with *two* independent variables being investigated, there are *three* null hypotheses.

H_{01}: retention interval is not a factor in the test score achieved,

H_{02}: age is not a factor in the test score achieved, and

H_{03}: the interaction between age and retention interval is not a factor in the test score achieved.

The extract above summarizes the results of the two-way analyses of variance which tested this set of hypotheses for each of the eight tests the sample were asked to complete. The main effects of the retention interval (H_{01}) were reported first. The layout has been changed slightly for ease of comprehension.

> Main effects of RI were significant for
>
> name recognition ($F(5,355) = 9.07, p < .001$);
>
> concept recognition ($F(5,355) = 18.57, p < .001$);
>
> fact verification specific ($F(5,355) = 2.41, p < .05$);
>
> grouping ($F(5,355) = 6.30, p < .001$);
>
> cued recall of names ($F(5,355) = 3.95, p < .001$); and for
>
> cued recall of concepts ($F(5,355) = 6.95, p < .001$).
>
> The effects of RI were not significant in the test of fact verification general nor in the test of experimental design
>
> (Ibid.)

The paragraph then goes on to report the main effects of age (H_{02}) and then the interaction effects (H_{03}). The concluding comment illustrates the importance of the two-way design, and one of its advantages over the simple one-way design. The one-way ANOVA which was used first to study the effect of age on test scores had suggested that age could be a factor in achievement on some types of test. However, as the researchers pointed out, age was highly correlated with the retention interval. In other words, the older students were also those with the longest gap since they had studied. The two-way ANOVA showed both that there was no interaction effect and that age appeared to be a less important factor than retention interval.

The analysis of variance approach can be used in much more complex ways in situations where researchers want to examine the effects of more than two independent variables at a time, or where they want to examine the effects on several *dependent* variables at the same time. In this latter situation, they would be using a modified form of analysis of variance termed multivariate analysis of variance or MANOVA for short. These forms of analysis are relatively uncommon in that the underlying statistical assumptions about the data which the techniques make, grow more demanding — and the interpretation of the results also becomes more complex and difficult.

STATS PIECE 14: ANALYSIS OF VARIANCE FOR MORE THAN TWO INDEPENDENT VARIABLES

Suppose researchers wish to test the relationship of four independent variables (A, B, C and D) with one dependent variable using an analysis of variance technique. Then the following effects would be tested, with fourteen different hypotheses involved. Suppose the dependent variable is (say) non-attendance at school. Then the researchers would be testing the following sets of hypotheses.

Main effects:

- variable A, H_{01}, variable A is not a factor in non-attendance at school
- variable B, H_{02}, variable B is not a factor in non-attendance at school
- variable C, H_{03}, variable C is not a factor in non-attendance at school
- variable D, H_{04}, variable D is not a factor in non-attendance at school.

First-order interactions:

- A/B, H_{05}, the interaction between A and B is not a factor in non-attendance at school
- A/C, H_{06}, the interaction between A and C is not a factor in non-attendance at school
- A/D, H_{07}, the interaction between A and D is not a factor in non-attendance at school
- B/C, H_{08}, the interaction between B and C is not a factor in non-attendance at school
- B/D, H_{09}, the interaction between B and D is not a factor in non-attendance at school
- C/D, H_{10}, the interaction between C and D is not a factor in non-attendance at school.

Second-order interactions:

- A/B/C, H_{11}, the interaction between A, B and C is not a factor in non-attendance at school
- A/B/D, H_{12}, the interaction between A, B and D is not a factor in non-attendance at school
- B/C/D, H_{13}, the interaction between B, C and D is not a factor in non-attendance at school.

Third-order interaction:

- A/B/C/D, H_{14}, the interaction between A, B, C and D is not a factor in non-attendance at school.

Residual variance:

In practice, the second- and third-order interaction terms are very difficult to interpret sensibly, unless the theory underlying the study makes specific predictions about them. Many analysts add them to the residual variance as a composite error term.

6.3 REGRESSION TECHNIQUES

The techniques discussed above enable us to explore the effects of more than one independent variable on a dependent variable, or (which is the same thing) to control statistically for the effects of extraneous variables. They have the advantage that they allow us to explore interaction effects as well as main effects in a fairly straightforward manner. Their weakness, however, is that they are cumbersome to use and/or difficult to interpret when the number of independent variables grows beyond about three or four. A second family of techniques, based around notions of correlation and regression, has been devised to overcome this problem.

In the third reading associated with this unit the analyses of variance show that age and retention interval both appear to have a significant effect on the scores achieved in certain tests. To extend the analysis the researchers carried out a form of multivariate analysis called *multiple regression*. You may recall that simple linear regression is a way of examining the extent to which one variable can be predicted by another. Multiple regression is a simple extension of the idea of linear regression to allow us to predict one variable from a combination of several others. The researchers examined the contribution of each of four different predictor variables (retention interval, age at retrieval, grade, and interest) to the total variance of each test score. However, it is possible to include more independent variables if this seems appropriate. The aim of researchers in using multiple regression is usually to try to develop a model (in the form of an equation) which can use information about a set of independent variables to predict the dependent variable as accurately as possible (Figure 16). The more of the variation in the dependent variable which the regression equation can explain, the more accurate will be the predictions. Unfortunately, in practice, there is usually a substantial amount of variance which is unaccounted for by regression models. This is termed the residual or the error variance.

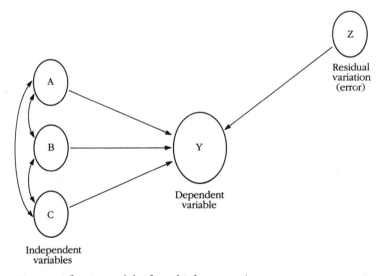

Figure 16 A model of multiple regression

The 'zero-order' effect of each variable — its effect by itself, ignoring the effects of other variables — is given by the correlation coefficient r. Remember that squaring r yields the proportion of variance explained for a pair of variables. Going back to the third reading if the four independent variables being examined as predictor variables were entirely independent of each other, we could just add the four proportions together to obtain total proportion of variance explained. However, if the four variables are correlated not just with the dependent variable but with each other as well, this means that we would be counting some of the variance explained *twice* or even more if we just add the proportions together (see shaded areas in Figure 17). In other words the total explained variance is less than the sum of the proportions. This point is shown visually in Figure 17, where the circles are the proportion of variance explained by each variable by itself, and the heavy line is the total proportion explained.

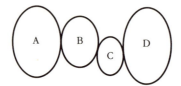

(a) Uncorrelated variables

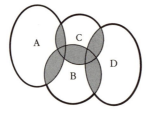

(b) Correlated variables

Figure 17 *Proportions of variance explained*

What multiple regression does is to assess the total proportion of variance explained by all the variables together, taking their correlation into account. The regression equation for predicting the amount of knowledge a student had retained using a single independent variable such as age would be, for example:

amount retained = $a + b \times$ (age) + error.

For all four variables, the multiple regression equation would be:

amount retained = $a + b_1 \times$ (age) + $b_2 \times$ (grade) + $b_3 \times$ (RI) + $b_4 \times$ (interest) + error.

The results are not presented as an equation, however, but as a series of summary statistics.

1. The overall prediction yields R, a multiple correlation coefficient. R^2, the coefficient of determination, is the proportion of variance explained overall. ('R' is used instead of 'r' because we are dealing with *multiple* correlation rather than simple correlation between *pairs* of variables. You came across r^2 in Section 5.2 as the coefficient of determination for a simple linear regression.)

2. The significance of R^2 will be tested, using an F-statistic, to see whether the overall level of prediction allows the rejection of the null hypothesis of no overall association (see Stats Piece 15).

3. Some computer programs will also test, again using the F-statistic, whether R is a significantly better predictor than the largest of the zero-order r values — in other words, whether anything is gained by adding in the extra independent variables.

4. For each variable, a beta coefficient will often be supplied (β_1, β_2, etc.). These are derived from the regression coefficients (b_1, b_2, etc.) by standardizing them (converting to z-scores), and they are also referred to as *standardized partial regression coefficients*. They estimate the independent contribution of each variable to the prediction, controlling for overlap with all the other variables in the equation. The larger this is, the larger the effect of that particular independent variable on the dependent variable.

5. Finally, this estimate is tested for significance (generally using Student's t-test). If the t is *not* significant, the prediction would be just as good if that variable were left out of the equation.

Therefore, a straightforward multiple regression analysis yields an overall estimate of variance explained (R^2), a test of its significance (the F-test), a test of whether each variable is contributing significantly (the t-tests), and possibly an estimate of each variable's *independent* effect (the β coefficients).

In the third reading, you will see that these statistics are summarized in Table 5 in the paper. For each of six tests the contribution of each variable to the overall variance is estimated (shown in columns headed v) and the results of the tests of their significances, in terms of their contribution to the overall prediction, are shown in the columns headed t.

STATS PIECE 15: USING F TO TEST THE SIGNIFICANCE OF R^2

The statistic used for assessing the statistical significance of R^2 and therefore of the fit of the regression line to the data, that is whether the regression line is a better predictor of Y-values than just using the mean, is the F-statistic. The null hypothesis is that, in the population, X and Y are not related, so that Y-values cannot be predicted from X-values. The correlation coefficient gives a measure of variance explained by the regression line, and the F-statistic tests the size of the ratio of this to the residual variance, to see if it is greater than we might reasonably expect in a sample from a population in which X and Y were not really associated.

If you check back to Stats Piece 10, you will recall that:

total variance = explained variance + residual variance.

In Table 13 this was written in analysis of variance terms as:

SS (total) = SS (between groups) + SS (within groups).

However, it can also be written in more general terms (see the first column of Table 13) as:

total sum of squares (TSS) = explained sum of square (ESS) + residual sum of squares (RSS).

Where we are looking at more than one independent variable, the coefficient of determination is written as R^2.

$$R^2 = \frac{ESS}{TSS} = 1 - \frac{RSS}{TSS}.$$

But remember from Stats Piece 9 that

$$F = \frac{\text{explained mean square}}{\text{residual mean square}}$$

$$= \frac{\text{explained sum of squares } (n - k)}{\text{residual sum of squares } (k - 1)}.$$

Then from these two equations it can be shown that:

$$F = \frac{R^2/k}{(1 - R^2)/(n - k - 1)}$$

where k is the number of groups.

Before leaving the topic of multiple linear regression, one variant which you are very likely to encounter in your reading is *stepwise* multiple regression. Here the variables are entered one at a time, starting with the one which has the largest effect, then the one which adds most to the prediction with the first variable already in the equation, then the one which adds most given that the first two are already in the equation, and so on until no other variable makes a significant contribution. The history of this process and whether the value of R rises significantly as each variable is entered would generally be reported, along with the statistics discussed above. A problem in interpreting stepwise analysis is that the first variable to enter the equation necessarily makes a disproportionately large contribution because it is treated initially as not correlated with any other variable; you need to inspect the β coefficients to see how much the influence of each variable *changes* as another enters the equation, which may be of interest in some studies.

Another 'trick' for estimating the importance of a given variable is to remove it from the final equation. Let us say we have an *R* value based on four independent variables. If we remove a particular variable from the equation and *R* becomes significantly smaller, then we know how much that variable is contributing to the prediction. If *R* does *not* drop significantly, then the prediction would be just as good without it.

Another variant of regression analysis is called *path analysis* (see Figure 18). If you can establish a logical 'causal order' to your independent variables, then you can look at their causal influence on each other as well as on the dependent variable. In Figure 18, for example, suppose that A, B and C were father's social class, mother's social class and level of education reached, predicting social class of child at age 25 (Y). The two 'parental' variables logically precede education and have a causal effect on it. (The two parental variables are probably correlated with each other — people tend to marry within social class more than they do outside it.) Now, education has only a direct effect on child's social class (the pathway from C to Y). Parental classes, however, have two ways of influencing child's social class — *directly* (A–Y and B–Y) and *indirectly* via education (A–C–Y and B–C–Y). By carrying out a series of regression analyses you can estimate the strength of all these pathways.

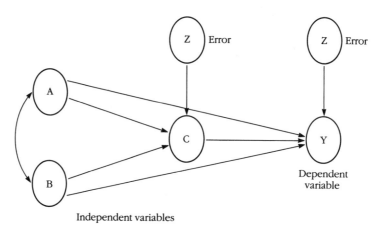

Figure 18 *A model of path analysis*

We have said all along that regression and correlation techniques are designed for numbers at the ratio level of measurement, may be used for interval or perhaps even ordinal data, but can never be used with nominal data. In general this is true. You could not, for example, use a variable of 'voting preference' (coded 1 = Labour, 2 = Conservative, 3 = other) in a regression equation, because the numbers do not mean anything — they are just labels. There is one exception to the rule, however: dichotomous data *can* be used in regression equations. A dichotomy is a variable with two values (e.g. gender: 1 = male, 2 = female). Although this is *interpreted* as a nominal variable — 'female' could not be said to be twice 'male' — it *behaves* like a ratio variable. The mean is interpretable — if a group has a mean gender score of 1.67, it is two-thirds female and one-third male — and so are the standard deviation and variance.

That being so, you can enter any variable as an independent variable in a regression equation and represent it as a dichotomy (or more than one). We might do this by re-coding. In the example above, for instance, 'voting preference' might be represented as Labour (1) vs Conservative (2), leaving out the 'others' altogether. Or, depending on the hypothesis to be tested, you might re-code it as major parties (codes 1 and 2) vs others (code 3). However, if you wish to preserve all the information, what you can do is to enter it as a series of *dummy variables* (dichotomies), thus:

Dummy 1: Labour (code 1) vs others (codes 2, 3)

Dummy 2: Conservative (code 2) vs others (codes 1, 3).

This preserves all the information:

if old code was 1, Dummy 1 is coded 1 and Dummy 2 is coded 0

if old code was 2, Dummy 1 is coded 0 and Dummy 2 is coded 1

if old code was 3, Dummy 1 is coded 0 and Dummy 2 is coded 0.

It is not good practice to use a dichotomy as *dependent* variable, however. Regression tries to build a continuous prediction line, minimizing residual deviation from it and finishing up with a random distribution of deviations along the line. With a dichotomy as dependent variable this process can never be very successful because the dependent variable can take only one of two values, not the continuous distribution which the prediction equation assumes. You will find analyses in the research literature which use a dichotomy as independent variable (particularly in the literature on social class) but it is none the less not good practice — a different kind of analysis is needed.

6.4 RELATED MULTIVARIATE APPROACHES

Log-linear analysis

With analysis of various techniques, we saw how the effects of independent variables on dependent variables could be tested. We also saw how multiple linear regression could be used to build predictive models and to measure the strength of the relationship between the dependent variable and the set of independent variables. This is achieved by using the coefficient of determination R^2 to identify the proportion of the total variation in the dependent variable which was explained by this set of variables. However, neither of these sets of techniques should be used with categorical level data from populations which do not have normal distributions and constant variance. In situations where the research problem involves categorical data — either where the researcher wishes to identify relationships between variables, and what their effect is on each other, or where a predictive model is wanted — then the analysis is likely to involve a technique known as *log-linear analysis*.

Researchers construct a multivariate contingency table, then investigate the relationship between the variables, treating *all* the variables used in the table as independent variables, with the dependent variables being the *number of cases* located in each cell of the contingency table. The linear model which is developed as a result of this analysis enables cell frequencies to be predicted. The better the model, the closer the predicted or expected frequency is to the observed frequency. The distinctive feature of this particular technique, and the one which gives the technique its name, is that the natural logs of the cell frequencies are used in the construction of the linear model.

The principle behind the construction of a log-linear model is very similar to that for chi-square in that the observed frequencies and the expected frequencies are compared cell by cell. Unlike chi-square, however, log-linear analysis enables researchers to explore higher order interaction effects from several different variables. Suppose, for example, that researchers wanted to study the possible relationship between the line of study students propose to choose and their gender. They might also hypothesize that social class and level of satisfaction with their studies might be associated. Using log-linear analysis, the researchers could test hypotheses about the effects of the variables on each other through examining the interaction of the variables — for instance, whether a second order interaction of social class and satisfaction with course exists, or whether a third order interaction of gender, satisfaction with course and social class contributes to the model.

Just as with multiple regression, the aim is to construct as simple a model as possible which will accurately predict the frequencies to be found in particular cells in the multi-way contingency table. You will have noticed the 'family connection' with analysis of variance in that the effects of particular variables can be tested through examining different orders of interaction and through testing individual terms (as we saw in Stats Piece 14).

One variation of log-linear analysis now enjoying some popularity is *logit analysis*. With log-linear analysis, all the variables are treated as independent variables with the cell frequencies being the dependent variables (i.e. the variable which is predicted by the other variables). However, logit models enable log-linear analysis to be used to examine the relationship between independent variables and a dependent dichotomous variable. So in our example we might have line of study having the two categories of arts and science as the dependent variable, with the other variables being the independent variables.

Discriminant analysis

A rather different form of analysis, but one still linked both to multiple regression and analysis of variance is discriminant analysis. Many social scientists see this as a very useful analytic tool in that it can be used both to predict the group to which a person or 'case' might belong on the basis of a set of characteristics which that person or case holds, and it can be used to identify which variables are most powerful in distinguishing between the members of different groups. Take, for example, juvenile crime. Researchers may have drawn together a range of socio-economic information about a sample of youngsters — some of whom may be consistent offenders, others who may be first offenders, and a third group with no known convictions. Discriminant analysis could be used by the researchers to identify which of the socio-economic data they held was most useful in discriminating between members of the three different groups. They could also devise a model in the form of an equation using the data they held to enable them to predict the group membership for other youngsters. This form of analysis clearly has many applications. It has been used in credit risk work, psychological testing, investigating effects of medical treatment, researching sentencing practices and studying voting intentions.

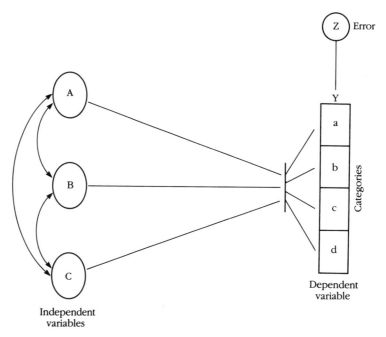

Figure 19 *A model of discriminant function analysis*

In Figure 19, no directions are indicated between the discriminating variables and the group categories. This is because the causation can be in either direction. If group membership is seen as being dependent on the variables, then the analysis is very closely related to multiple regression except that the dependent variable (the groups) is a nominal (also called categorical) level, variable. However, if the values of the discriminating variables are seen as being dependent on the group to which the case or individual belongs, then the analysis can be seen as closely associated with analysis of variance. One example of the latter situation would include research into sex differences in behaviour or attitudes, where the behaviour measures might be hypothesized as being dependent on the gender of the individual. Another example might be a study of the effects of 'setting' in schools on a range of pupil self-esteem and achievement measures.

The form which the model would take would be:

$$F = u_0 + u_1 X_1 + u_2 X_2 + u_3 X_3$$

where F is the function or the discriminant score for a particular case or member of the sample. The size of this score would determine the case's membership of a particular group. The Xs represent the values for that case on each of the three discriminating variables in this model, and the u values are the standardized coefficients which have been calculated from the data set which determine how much each variable X contributes to the overall discriminant score.

The output which will be reported includes:

1. A statistic assessing the significance of the prediction — whether using the independent variables to predict in which category each case should fall improves the prediction at all over chance. The most commonly used statistic is Wilks' Λ (lambda), which counts in the opposite direction from most of the statistics we have considered in this unit: a value of 1 means no difference from chance, and a value of 0 means perfect prediction.

2. An indication of which variables contributed to the prediction and by how much.

3. A 'hits and misses' table, tabulating actual category against predicted category and giving the percentage correctly classified by the prediction equation.

There are, as always, some limitations and difficulties associated with using this technique. There are the statistical assumptions which must be met, such as that the discriminating variables must be interval level and that groups are drawn from populations with normal distributions on the discriminating variables. There are also practical problems with interpreting the output. For example, the model which is constructed from one data set may not be as efficient at prediction with a different data set, as each new case can slightly modify the coefficients. A good model needs testing with a number of different data sets. Also, for a model to be useful the variables it incorporates as discriminating variables do need to be well chosen initially.

One relatively new technique which makes fewer statistical demands on the data is logistic regression for dependent variables which take only two values. With logistic regression the probability of an event occurring is estimated. As with both discriminant analysis and multiple regression, stepwise entry of variables into the equation is allowed. The equation which can be constructed from the output gives a statistic which is the estimated probability of an event. Normally, if the probability is less than 0.5, then the event is predicted not to occur.

6.5 FACTOR ANALYSIS

Finally, for completeness' sake, we ought to think briefly about *factor analysis*. We shall not go into the complexities of what can easily turn into a *very* complex topic, but you may find it useful, when reading research reports which use it, to be familiar with some of the basic concepts.

Factor analysis works, like many of the analyses in this unit, by trying to fit a model to data in such a way as to minimize squared deviations from a set of predicted values. However, it is used for a different purpose from the other analyses in this unit. It *can* be used for hypothesis-testing, for example, testing whether it is reasonable to say that a set of data is *unidimensional* (can be adequately described by locating data points on a single dimension). More often it is used for simplifying complex data by finding the minimum number of dimensions that can be used to describe them without leaving a large amount of the variance unexplained. For example, you might have ratings of a person on a large number of dimensions (amount of smiling, friendliness, openness, amiability, likelihood of stealing, likelihood of lying, number of times in trouble with the police ...), and you might want to group these into a smaller number of summary variables (warmth, law-abiding nature ...) (see Figure 20). Factor analysis enables you to do this with some rigour, and to identify the items which do not fit any of the summary variables and which should be discarded.

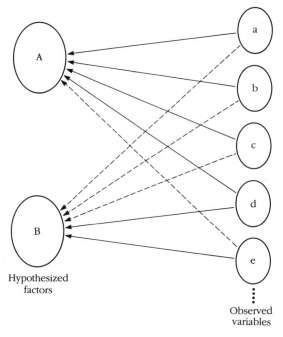

Figure 20 *A model of factor analysis*

The first element in a factor analysis is a *principal components analysis*. This creates as many components as there were variables in the original data set. However, it seeks (a bit like a stepwise multiple regression done backwards) to make some of these components account for far more of the variance than others. The first component will attempt to explain as much of the variance as possible (like a regression line through a multidimensional space); the second will try to account for as much as possible of the variance which remains; and so on. Thus you finish up with a set of components of which the first few (or even just the first one) account for most of the variance in the data set, while the rest account for only trivial amounts.

Many researchers stop at this point and report on the 'important' components (selected 'by eye' or using one of a range of more rigorous methods). A full-blown factor analysis involves one more stage, however, in which the lines are *rotated* through the data-space to improve the fit of those factors which are retained from the principle compenentos analysis. This process is illustrated in a simple way in Figure 21. Figure 21(a) illustrates what might be the two major components of a

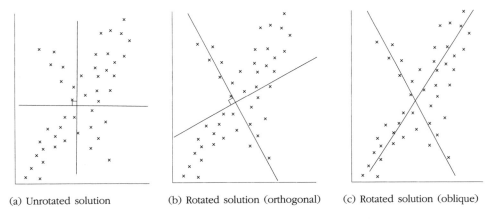

(a) Unrotated solution (b) Rotated solution (orthogonal) (c) Rotated solution (oblique)

Figure 21 *Rotation in factor analysis*

principal components analysis; the data points can be located by reference to these two lines, and no third dimension is needed to establish where each data point is. The two components are independent of each other (not correlated), so the lines are shown as at right angles to each other. Figure 21(b) shows an *orthogonal rotation*; the two factors remain uncorrelated, but they have been rotated round to fit the data points better (i.e. to minimize squared deviations from the two lines). Most researchers use orthogonal (uncorrelated) factors because they are interested in the number of *independent* factors that can usefully be extracted from the data. Other forms of rotation are possible, however, and Figure 21(c) illustrates an *oblique rotation,* with the two lines *no longer at right angles* to each other. This fits the data better, but the two factors are correlated with each other, which can sometimes make interpretation more difficult.

A final point to note is that factor analysis is an interpretative art as much as a rigorous statistical procedure. You may be able to use statistical decision-making techniques to determine the number of factors, but what they are to be called (i.e. what they *mean*) must be determined by the researcher and the reader. Suppose, for example, that we had three factors loaded as in Table 18. The first is fairly easy to label: call it 'warmth' or 'friendliness'. The second looks like 'honesty' or 'law-abiding nature', but this could be because of what we have chosen to record. (If we had also taken measures of 'risk-taking' and 'preference for challenge', for example, and they were loaded under this factor, then we might want to call it something like 'caution' or 'staying out of trouble'.) The third is very difficult to interpret at all, unless as a measure of ability with paper-and-pencil tests. In other words, factor analysis uses computers for what they do best — rapid, large-scale calculation — and leaves the burden of interpretation with the researcher.

Table 18 Three hypothetical factors and their constituent variables

Factor 1	Factor 2	Factor 3
Ratings of friendliness	Number of times in trouble with police	Intelligence test score
Ratings of warmth	Ratings of honesty	Neurotism inventory score
Ratings of openness	Ratings of likelihood of stealing	Extroversion inventory score
Number of smiles in test situation		

7 FINAL COMMENTS

At the beginning of the unit I commented that, after having worked through the whole unit, you should be in a position to read critically and understand a wider range of research papers and reports. The particular type of research paper or report I had in mind was, of course, those reporting the findings of quantitative research.

ACTIVITY 14

For Activity 1 you were asked to scan the three readings associated with this unit, making notes of those parts you found particularly difficult to handle or interpret. You should now go back to your notes and check off those problems which have been clarified.

You should find that at least some of the queries you noted before starting this unit no longer present a problem. However, it would be surprising if you did not still have a number of points which you felt were not clear. With a topic such as analysis, it can be necessary to read and re-read texts a number of times before ideas 'click'. However, you've shown perseverance in getting this far with the unit!, so you can rest assured that over time the issues we've been discussing will become clearer. One of the best ways of moving forward at this point is actually to carry out some of your own analysis and interpret it. Both the next activity and TMA 07 will help you here.

ACTIVITY 15

The final activity in this unit is designed to prepare you for TMA 07. You should listen to the audio-cassette programme 'Analysing structured data' and carry out the computer analyses which it suggests. You will also need the notes to accompany this cassette which are in the Audio-visual Handbook.

You may also find it useful to read some new journal articles reporting quantitative research — perhaps chosen from your own field of interest — remembering to refer back to the unit to refresh your understanding of the terms and approaches being used. With further practice in reading and critical reflection your appreciation of the ways in which researchers use the quantitative analysis tools available to them will grow and deepen.

ANSWERS TO ACTIVITIES

ACTIVITY 2

- *Nominal*: gender, town of birth, political allegiance, educational level (coded 'vocational', 'academic', 'others').

- *Ordinal*: grade, social class, intelligence score, educational level (coded by highest qualification achieved).

- *Interval*: temperature, time of day, musical pitch, educational level (coded by year-group at school).

- *Ratio*: age, retention interval, income, educational level (coded by years of schooling).

From the readings I picked:

1 gender — clearly nominal;

2 grade — superficially an interval variable, but we cannot be sure that the intervals are equal, so better treated as ordinal;

3 age — clearly a ratio variable (but see below); and

4 retention interval — clearly ratio.

Searching for other examples, I thought of place of birth (Manchester, London, Birmingham, ...) and political allegiance (Labour, Conservative, Liberal ...) as examples of nominal variables. The underlying variables could be of a higher level in both cases — 'place of birth' could be coded in terms of how far north it was in the British Isles, for example, or political allegiance in terms of degree of radicalism. As they stand, however, the categories are just descriptive names.

For ordinal variables I had social class and intelligence score — neither can be shown unequivocally, as I argued in the text, to have equal intervals between scores or codes. For interval variables I had temperature, time of day and musical pitch, all measures where the intervals are equal but any zero on the scale is purely arbitrary. For an unequivocally ratio variable I picked income.

The major problem is that something which is of a ratio nature in itself can be degraded by the coding (age, coded as 'older', 'middle', or 'younger', is ordinal). I have included educational level in all four categories depending on its coding.

ACTIVITY 3

You can see from Table 2 that the greatest spread of ages occurs among the former students who last studied the course either 6 or 9 years ago (where RI equals 77 and 113 months). Figure 22 shows how the age distributions might look for the group with the greatest standard deviation as compared to the group with the smallest standard deviation. The greatest difference is between the group who last studied 9 years and 3 months ago (RI = 113) who have a mean age of 53.3 with a standard deviation of 11.9 years, and those who last studied the course only 3 months ago who have a mean age of 39.6 years, with a standard deviation of 8.1 years.

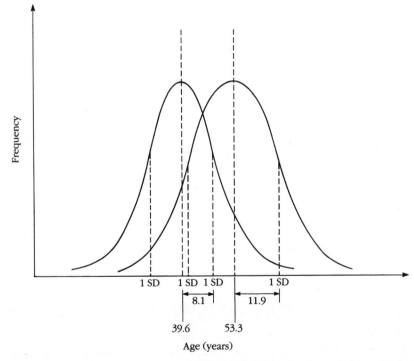

Figure 22 Mean age and standard deviation for RI = 3 and 113 months

ACTIVITY 4

Because the data are given as percentages, the reader can see at a glance the extent to which the three age groups differ in terms of their distribution across different retention intervals.

Interpretation for the casual reader would probably be easier if there was a final column to the table on the right-hand side showing the total frequency for each of the age groups and indicating that these were the bases on which the row percentages were based. Table 19 shows how the addition of a final column to Table 4 and the inclusion of per cent signs could aid its interpretation.

Table 19 Percentages of young, middle-aged and elderly subjects distributed across retention intervals (amended)

Age		Retention intervals in years						Total
		0.25–2	3–4	5–6	7–8	9–10	11–12	
Young	%	41	22	23	7	4	3	100
Middle-aged	%	12	15	29	18	14	12	100
Elderly	%	4	11	12	16	26	30	100

(Source: adapted from Cohen et al., 1992b, Table 1a)

We can see quite easily that the three distributions are each a very different shape. The mode for the 'young' group is the 0.25–2 interval, with 41 per cent in it (Figure 23a); the mode for the 'middle-aged' group is the 5–6 year interval with 29 per cent of the group (Figure 23b); and the mode for the 'elderly' group in the 11–12 year interval which contains 30 per cent of the group (Figure 23c).

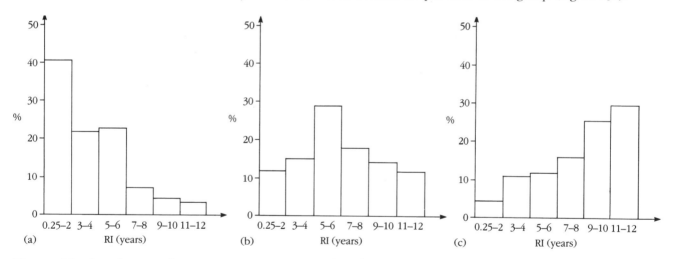

Figure 23 Distribution of age across retention intervals: (a) young, (b) middle-aged and (c) elderly

What we have very clearly is a *positively skewed* distribution (the 'young' group); a *normal* distribution (the 'middle-aged' group); and a *negatively skewed* distribution (the 'elderly' group).

ACTIVITY 5

The first extract reads easily, but has relatively little information in it. The one clear statistical term the writer uses is 'percentages'. This gives precise information about data retention. The piece is talking about recent graduates *as a group*. In fact the author of the piece is talking about average or mean scores, but this is implied rather than stated. Nor is any mention made of the variability of the scores among the 'recent graduates'.

UNIT 19/20 ANALYSIS OF STRUCTURED DATA

The second extract conveys a greater amount of information, together with more detail. Here the authors refer to averages but without explicitly mentioning means. Percentages are again used, with comparisons over time being made. Mention of variability is made, but this appears to refer more to the lack of smoothness of the trend than to the variability of individual scores about the mean. Finally a reference to the significance of the data is made. This term comes from inferential statistics rather than descriptive statistics. You will cover such issues in Section 4.

ACTIVITY 6

Remember that a Type 1 error occurs if the null hypothesis H_0 is rejected when in fact it is true. If the researchers want to minimize the possibility of this occurring, then they will want to minimize α. Consider the following example.

Suppose we have a situation where assessors or examiners are judging someone's competence in (say) plumbing. The null hypothesis H_0 might be stated as follows: the student has not displayed the necessary competence to practice as a qualified plumber. If this null hypothesis is true, then a wrong rejection of it would mean that someone who was not competent on a key skill would be free to practice on an unsuspecting public. From the public's perspective, the aim should be to minimize the possibility of a wrong rejection of this hypothesis. In other words they would want Type 1 errors minimized. In contrast the unfortunate candidates would feel strongly that emphasis should be given to minimizing Type 2 errors; in other words to minimizing the possibility of not rejecting H_0 when it is false. Otherwise people who *were* competent might be wrongly assessed as not competent.

Researchers would want to minimize the possibility of Type 1 error in any case where the outcome of rejecting H_0, when it was in fact true, could lead to gross inequity or to great wastage of resources. Research on gender differences in intelligence or educatability, for example, requires a very high 'standard of proof', because to base policy on such supposed differences, if they do not in fact exist, would be most unjust. On the other hand, we should also want a high standard of proof that a new medical procedure was indisputably more effective than existing alternatives, if it were also vastly more expensive.

ACTIVITY 7

In Table 3(a), the number of rows r is 3, while the number of columns c is 4. The number of degrees of freedom is therefore:

$$df = (r - 1) \times (c - 1)$$

$$df = (3 - 1) \times (4 - 1)$$

$$= 2 \times 3 = 6.$$

ACTIVITY 8

Let us look at the extract laid out a little more clearly.

> By χ^2 the distribution of age groups is significantly different for all these variables:
> RI (χ^2 (10) = 98.42, $p < .0001$);
> grade (χ^2 (6) = 18.40, $p < .005$); and
> interest (χ^2 (4) = 10.90, $p < .02$).
>
> (Cohen *et al.*, 1992b)

The conclusions in the extract are based on the information shown in Tables 1(a), 1(b) and 1(c) in the third reading (reproduced as Tables 4, 3(a) and 3(b) in this unit). First I checked the degrees of freedom for each of the tables as follows.

For Table 4, age by RI, $r = 3$ and $c = 6$, therefore the degrees of freedom are calculated as:

$$df = (3 - 1) \times (6 - 1)$$
$$= 2 \times 5 = 10.$$

For Table 3(a), age by grade, $r = 3$ and $c = 4$, therefore the degrees of freedom are calculated as:

$$df = (3 - 1) \times (4 - 1)$$
$$= 2 \times 3 = 6.$$

For Table 3(b), age by interest, $r = 3$ and $c = 3$, therefore the degrees of freedom are calculated as:

$$df = (3 - 1) \times (3 - 1)$$
$$= 2 \times 2 = 4.$$

I then checked each of the χ^2 for the appropriate degrees of freedom against Table 5 in the Statistics Handbook.

For age by RI (Table 4), I got for a χ^2 of 98.42 with 10 df, $p < .001$. The research team reported $p < .0001$, but our tables do not give this level of detail. Nevertheless, it is clear that the difference being tested is highly significant, with a less than one in 1,000 likelihood of having occurred by chance.

For age by grade (Table 3a), for a χ^2 of 18.40 with 6 df, I got $p < .01$. This figure reported in the reading is $p < .005$. Again, our tables do not carry the information for p at .005, but nevertheless, our figure and the published figure do not contradict each other.

For age by interest (Table 3b), for a χ^2 of 10.90 with 4 df, I got a $p < .05$. The published figure was $p < .02$, but for this, χ^2 would have to have been 11.67 or more. Although the difference in the p values would not affect the conclusions drawn, I decided to check out the figures with the researchers to see what they thought had happened. They then re-ran the table on the computer and got a slightly different set of figures from the ones originally recorded, with $\chi^2 = 13.74$ at 4 df and $p < .01$. They also re-ran the other two χ^2 figures again, and marginally different values emerged. After examining both sets of statistics, the researchers concluded that the differences were due to working with different computer software packages.

The three sets of χ^2 figures which were achieved using the same research data, but using the STATSVIEW package for the analysis, were:

RI, $\chi^2 = 97.596$ with 10 df, $p < .0001$

grade, $\chi^2 = 21.576$ with 6 df, $p < .01$

interest, $\chi^2 = 13.746$ with 4 df, $p < .01$

This slight discrepancy in the values illustrates well why it is always worth checking the statistics even in published papers. In this instance, the re-run revealed no substantive differences and the research conclusions stand.

ACTIVITY 9

Table 20 Calculation of χ^2 from Table 11

Gender	Population %	Sample %	Sample frequency (observed)	Expected frequency	$O - E$	$\dfrac{(O - E)^2}{E}$
Male	49.0	52.4	786	735	51	2601/735 = 3.54
Female	51.0	47.6	714	765	(51)[a]	2601/765 = 3.4
Total	100.0	100.0	1,500	1,500		$\chi^2 = 6.94$

[a] Figure in parentheses indicates a negative number.

The 'sample' column of Table 20 shows the 'observed' figures, i.e. the distribution between genders that was actually achieved. The 'population' column shows the distribution we would expect the sample to have. The $O - E$ column shows the difference between the figures that were actually observed in the sample, and the figures which would be expected for that size sample if they matched the population distribution. The final column shows the χ^2 calculation.

As regards the degrees of freedom, we have only one column of observed data, and two rows, so we have $(r - 1)$ degrees of freedom where $r = 2$, therefore $(2 - 1) = 1$ df.

Looking up a χ^2 value of 6.94 with 1 df in Table 5 in the Statistics Handbook, we find that the likelihood of a value of 6.94 for χ^2 at 1 df occurring by chance is less than .01, which is less than one in 100. The null hypothesis of 'no difference' may therefore safely be rejected, and we can assert that the sample does differ significantly from the population in respect of gender.

ACTIVITY 10

Because the researchers only want to test whether the mean of one group is *larger* than the mean of the other group, then they would need to use a *one-tailed* test.

The null hypothesis H_0 would be that the mean for women (u_w) was less than or equal to the mean for men (u_m).

This can be written as

$H_0: u_w \leq u_m$.

We know that $t = 2$ and we have 30 df. From Table 3 in the Statistics Handbook, reading for a one-tailed test with 30 df, $t \geq 1.697$ is significant at the .05 level (one-tailed) and $p < .05$.

If α is set at 0.05, α is greater than p ($\alpha > p$), so H_0 can be rejected. In other words we are saying that there is a less than 5 per cent probability that the difference in scores have arisen by chance. However, if α is set at 0.01, then α is less than p ($\alpha < p$), and we would *not* reject the null hypothesis. In other words we are saying that there is a greater than 1 per cent probability that the difference in scores could have arisen by chance.

ACTIVITY 12

The extract is summarizing the results of an analysis of variance (ANOVA). A series of pairs of variables is being investigated: namely retention interval (RI) and name recognition; RI and concept recognition; RI and fact verification, and so on. Remember that F is the ratio of the estimated variance based on the variation in means between the different groups and the estimated variance based on the variation in the measure within groups. In order to interpret F, its significance needs to be determined. The p value gives the likelihood of a particular measure of F for the two given degrees of freedom occurring by chance. So the first part of the extract: 'Main effects of RI were significant for name recognition ($F(5,355) = 9.07$, $p < .001$)' is saying that the likelihood of getting a measure of 9.07 for F with 5 degrees of freedom for the explained (or between-groups) variation (V_1) and 355 degrees of freedom for the residual (or within groups) variation (V_2) by chance is less than one in 1,000.

Similarly the next part of the extract ' ... concept recognition ($F(5,355) = 18.57$, $p < .001$)' is saying that the likelihood of getting scores for concept recognition by chance which have a distribution giving a measure of 18.57 for F with 5 degrees of freedom for the explained variation (V_1) and 355 degrees of freedom for the residual variation (V_2) is less than one in 1,000.

All the variables listed in the extract have F values which are seen as unlikely to have arisen by chance for the particular number of degrees of freedom given.

FURTHER READING

Quantitative Applications in the Social Sciences, A Sage University Paper Series, Newbury Park, Sage.

This series of methodological works provides introductory explanations and demonstrations of data analysis techniques applicable to the social sciences.

REFERENCES

Cohen, G., Stanhope, N. and Conway, M. (1992a) 'How long does education last? Very long term retention of cognitive psychology', *The Psychologist*, vol. 5, pp.57–60 (reproduced in Offprints Booklet 4).

Cohen, G., Stanhope, N. and Conway, M. (1992b) 'Age differences in the retention of knowledge by young and elderly students', *British Journal of Developmental Psychology*, vol. 10, Part 2, pp.153–64 (reproduced in Offprints Booklet 4).

Conway, M., Cohen, G. and Stanhope, N. (1991) 'On the very long-term retention of knowledge acquired through formal education: twelve years of cognitive psychology', *Journal of Experimental Psychology*, vol. 120, no. 4, pp.395–409.

Electronics World and Wireless World (1992) 'How non-volatile is brainpower?', Research Notes, May, p.360 (reproduced in Offprints Booklet 4).

ACKNOWLEDGEMENTS

Grateful acknowledgement is made to the following sources for permission to reproduce material in these units:

TABLES

Table 2: Conway, M., Cohen, G. and Stanhope, N. (1991) 'On the very long-term retention of knowledge acquired through formal education', *Journal of Experimental Psychology*, vol. 120, no. 4, December, copyright 1991 by the American Psychological Association. Reprinted by permisssion; Tables 3, 4 and 12: Cohen, G., Stanhope, N. and Conway, M. (1992) 'Age differences in the retention of knowledge by young and elderly students', *British Journal of Developmental Psychology*, vol. 10, Part 2, © 1992 British Psychological Society.

UNIT 21 CRITICAL ANALYSIS OF TEXT

Prepared for the Course Team by Victor Jupp

CONTENTS

Associated study materials		**102**
1	**Introduction**	**103**
2	**Documents, texts and discourses**	**104**
	2.1 Types of document	105
	2.2 The use of documents	109
3	**Traditions in documentary analysis**	**110**
	3.1 The positivist and interpretative uses of documents	111
4	**Critical social research**	**112**
	4.1 Critical analysis of documents	113
	4.2 Discourse analysis	114
	4.3 Case study 1: a proposal for critical analysis	115
	4.4 Case study 2: critical analysis of a public document	117
	4.5 Case study 3: critical analysis of decision making	119
	4.6 Case study 4: critical analysis of a research report	120
5	**Conclusion**	**120**
Answer to activity		**121**
References		**122**
Acknowledgement		**123**

ASSOCIATED STUDY MATERIALS

Reader, Chapter 4, 'The elements of critical social science', by Brian Fay.

Reader, Chapter 5, 'Traditions in documentary analysis', by Victor Jupp and Clive Norris.

Offprints Booklet 2, 'The origins of crime: the Cambridge Study in Delinquent Development', by David Farrington (reading associated with the audio-cassette).

Offprints Booklet 4, 'The telephone rings: long-term imprisonment', by Mike Fitzgerald.

Offprints Booklet 4, extracts from *Offending Women*, by Anne Worrall.

Audio-cassette 2, Side 2, 'A technical and critical analysis of a research report'.

1 INTRODUCTION

This unit is concerned with the use of documents in social research. The range of documents upon which social scientists have drawn includes diaries, letters, essays, personal notes, biographies and autobiographies, institutional memoranda and reports, and governmental pronouncements as in Green Papers, White Papers and Acts of Parliament. This list might give the impression that researchers are exclusively concerned with non-quantitative (sometimes called qualitative) documentary sources. However, this is not necessarily the case. As we shall see later in this unit, and especially in the associated audio-cassette, they are also interested in the way in which quantitative data are collected, assembled and analysed in order to reach conclusions.

Throughout this course a range of analytical strategies has been introduced. Some of these are structured and formal (as, say, in the analysis of experimental data) and others are less so; some strategies are founded on the principles of statistical analysis, whereas others follow the traditions and practices of qualitative research. Analytical strategies associated with structured and less structured data, and with quantitative and qualitative analyses, have found expression within the documentary tradition. Although these strands will all be represented in this unit, the main emphasis will be upon *critical analysis* of documents. The reason for this is that other styles of research (e.g. surveys, experimental) have already been covered in the course, as have other sources of data (e.g. interviews, observation). The unit brings together a distinct methodological approach — the *critical* — with particular forms of data — *documents*. (It should be recognized, however, that critical research is not exclusive to, and extends beyond the use of, documents.)

It is important to distinguish 'criticism', in its everyday usage, and 'critical analysis' as used by social scientists. The former usually refers to an evaluation which is negative, censorious or fault-finding. Critical analysis in social science involves an examination of the assumptions which underpin any account (say, in a document) and a consideration of what other possible aspects are concealed or ruled out. It can also involve moving beyond the documents themselves to encompass a critical analysis of the institutional and social structures within which such documents are produced. For example, one of the readings associated with this unit — that by Anne Worrall in Offprints Booklet 4 — is concerned with the assumptions about femininity which are found in probation reports about women offenders which are produced, and acted upon, in the criminal justice system in the UK. As with criticism in its everyday usage, critical analyses can involve being censorious or fault-finding, perhaps in terms of rejecting in-built assumptions of documents or seeking to overturn institutions or systems within which they are produced. However, this is not a necessary part of critical analysis.

In the main, this unit is concerned with 'reading about' documentary and textual analysis, although the emphasis switches to 'doing' documentary and textual analysis in the associated audio-cassette. The aims of the unit are as follows. The first seven aims involve 'reading about' documentary analysis; the final aim involves 'doing' critical analysis:

1 To identify and illustrate the range of documents used in social scientific research. The distinction between documents and texts will be made.

2 To contrast documentary analysis, as a method, with other forms of research covered in the course (such as survey and experimental methods).

3 To examine the influence of theoretical perspectives on documentary analysis.

4 In doing so, to distinguish three broad methodological approaches: the positivist, the interpretative and the critical.

5 To focus especially on critical analysis, including discourse analysis.

6 To emphasize that such critical analysis involves using documents as objects of research as opposed to resources within research.

7 To illustrate the critical analysis of a range of texts.

8 To carry out a critical analysis of a report based upon survey findings, and, in doing so, to distinguish the questions which a 'critical' analyst would ask from those which would be asked in an evaluation of the same report from a 'technical' point of view. This aim will be addressed primarily in the audio-cassette associated with this unit.

In comparison with some other sections of the course, this unit makes much greater reference to theoretical approaches. This is because the critical analysis of text, which is the main theme of the unit, makes much more obvious and explicit use of theoretical concepts and ideas than some other approaches (e.g. survey research which can often collect data without explicit reference to theory). Indeed, as will be emphasized throughout Section 4, the distinction between theorizing and empirical research is not one that is readily accepted by those who engage in critical analysis. Some of the concepts and ideas may seem rather abstract and complex, especially if this is your first encounter with critical analysis. It is for this reason that you should spend time gaining a firm understanding of them.

2 DOCUMENTS, TEXTS AND DISCOURSES

Scott (1990) has defined a document as a written text:

> Writing is the making of symbols representing words, and involves the use of a pen, pencil, printing machine or other tool for inscribing the message on paper, parchment or some other material medium.
>
> (Scott, 1990, p.12)

For Scott, the archetypal document is text that is handwritten or printed on paper. However, he recognizes that other media may also be bearers of text. For instance, gravestones are not documents, but they do carry texts, and the inscriptions on gravestones can be treated in the same way as if they were written on paper. In the same way, cell walls are not documents, but when inscribed with protests against prison conditions, or with political statements about the penal system, they can be viewed as such. Similarly, the extensive use of computers and word processors means that we should treat 'files' and 'documents' stored on tape and disks as documents suitable for analysis.

In short then, this unit adopts the distinction between document, as being the medium on which the message is stored, and text, the message that is conveyed through the symbols which constitute writing.

Documents can have a number of features. For example, they may be made up exclusively of written words, or they may include statistics, as in a survey research report. Documents may refer to particular individuals, as with school records and reports about pupils, or may concern more 'macro' issues, as with one of Her Majesty's Inspectorate Reports on the physical state of our schools. Further, documents may refer to contemporary events and issues, as in the case of newspaper reporting of a prison riot, for example, or they may relate to past events and issues, as in a nineteenth-century report on conditions in British prisons. Finally, documents may have been produced for purposes other than social research but nonetheless be of interest to researchers, in which case they are sometimes termed 'unobtrusive' measures' (Webb et al., 1966): 'An unobstrusive measure of observation is any method of observation that directly removes the observer from the set of interactions or events being studied' (Denzin, 1978, p.256). One rationale for the use of such measures is the belief that the effects of the observer on the data — the reactive effects discussed in earlier units — are reduced, thereby improving internal validity. Unobtrusive measures can derive from a number of sources, such as simple observations of behaviour without the individuals concerned knowing, or physical traces of behaviour left behind by individuals, and can also include documents. An example of the latter would be institutional memoranda, produced as a normal part of bureaucratic functioning but to which the social scientist can gain access in order to study key aspects of institutional processes. Punch (1985), for example, has outlined the use of police organizational records to study corruption amongst officers working in a red-light district of Amsterdam. The problem with the use of unobtrusive measures to study a sensitive issue such as police corruption is that access is vigorously denied by those who have interests in doing so.

In other instances, documents may be solicited deliberately and explicitly by social researchers and may even be produced by them, in which case they cannot be treated as unobtrusive measures. This is the case with many life histories, as outlined in Section 2.1 below. It is also true of detailed interviews which are recorded and transcribed by social scientists for subsequent analysis. For example, in Section 4 we examine the way in which data from the records and reports of probation officers, magistrates, solicitors and psychiatrists, and from transcriptions of detailed interviews with them, are used to examine decision making regarding women offenders.

There is one further term which deserves consideration in this section, namely *discourse*. The dictionary definition of discourse refers to talk, conversation and dissertation. Within social science it takes on a wider meaning as a result of its close association with a particular theoretical and methodological position which is covered in detail in Section 4.2, namely discourse analysis, one variant of what is described as critical analysis of text. As with documents and texts, discourses are concerned with communication. However, as Worrall points out, discourse goes much further than that 'to embrace all aspects of a communication — not only its content, but its author (who says it?), its authority (on what grounds?), its audience (to whom?), its objective (in order to achieve what?)' (Worrall, 1990, p.8).

Discourse encompasses sets of ideas, statements or knowledge which are dominant at a particular time among particular sets of people (e.g. 'expert professionals') and which are held in relation to other sets of individuals (e.g. patients or offenders). Such knowledge, ideas and statements provide explanations of what is problematic about the patients or offenders, why it is problematic and what should be done about it. In providing authority for some explanations, other forms of explanation are excluded. Implicit in the use of such knowledge is the application of power. In some instances, discourses may be viewed as imposed by professionals on clients but this is not necessarily the case. Discourses really come into their own when the client, for whatever reason and by whatever means, shares the professional's analysis of the problem and the means of addressing it. As indicated earlier, discourse involves all forms of communication, including talk and conversation. In the latter, however, it is not restricted exclusively to verbalized propositions, but can include ways of seeing, categorizing and reacting to the social world as in everyday practices, such as policing practices. Its relevance to this unit is that discourse can also be text expressed through the medium of documents.

2.1 TYPES OF DOCUMENT

A wide range of documents has been used in social research, including the following:

Life histories

The life history is similar to a biography or autobiography and is a means by which an individual provides a written record of his or her own life in his or her own terms. It can include a descriptive summary of life events and experiences and also an account of the social world from the subject's point of view. There is no concern with whether the account is 'right' or 'wrong'; if a subject sees the world in a particular way then that way is, for that person, 'right'. The examination of social perspectives and images is often a forerunner to the analysis of social actions, the assumption being that actions are underpinned by the way in which the social world is interpreted by actors.

Life histories may be written by the subject or by a second party, often a social scientist. A major landmark in the development of life history as a method was Thomas and Znaniecki's *The Polish Peasant in Europe and America*, volume one of which comprises a 300-page life history of a Polish emigré to Chicago in the early part of the twentieth century (Thomas and Znaniecki, 1958; first published in 1918–20). It provides an account, not only of life in an American city at that time, but also of the way in which it was experienced by the immigrant. Following Thomas and Znaniecki's work, the life history became an important element in what was known as the Chicago School of Sociology of the 1930s which focused especially on the problems of urban life.

Another important example of life history within the Chicago School was Clifford Shaw's *The Jack Roller* (Shaw, 1930), the story of Stanley, an adolescent boy whom Shaw met in prison where Stanley had been sent for 'jack rolling' (an activity akin to what we would now call mugging). It tells, in graphic detail, of Stanley's early upbringing and his years in various institutions before living on the streets and eventually becoming a jack roller. This was one of several life histories which led Shaw to formulate ideas about the transmission of criminal attitudes and values. This is illustrative of the way in which the collection and analysis of life history data can lead to formulation of social theory.

The diary

The diary has been used by both psychologists and sociologists but for different types of analysis. For example, the psychologist Allport focused on diaries as the prime means of uncovering the dynamics, structure and functioning of mental life (Allport, 1942). Also, Luria (1972) used diaries, among other accounts, to explore the experience of brain damage, leading to short-term memory loss. The sociologist Oscar Lewis (1959) used diaries to assemble data about the economy, lifestyle and daily activities of individuals in poor Mexican families. More recently, the diary has been used to gain insights into physical conditions and constraints of imprisonment, and individuals' subjective experiences, reactions and responses to them, as, for example, in Boyle's chronicling of his life in a number of Scottish prisons (Boyle, 1984). In a more formal sense, diaries can be used as part of survey methods, as in the National Food Survey outlined in Unit 9, in which families are asked to list their food intake over a period of one week.

Newspapers and magazines

The use of newspapers has been central in what is usually referred to as media analysis. Media analysis has several interests, one of which is an examination of the way in which stereotypes of categories of people or types of action are created, reinforced and amplified with wide-ranging consequences for those people and actions. For example, newspapers have been used to examine the portrayal of folk devils such as 'mods' and 'rockers' (Cohen, 1972), and the creation and career of the label and stereotype of 'mugger' in the British press (Hall *et al.*, 1978). Another example is Pearson's *Hooligan: A History of Respectable Fears* (1983) which relies heavily on nineteenth-century copies of the magazine *Punch* to examine the historical portrayal of the 'hooligan' and also to question the popular assertion that hooliganism is a recent phenomenon. Pearson notes that politicians of whatever decade often enlist a '20-year rule' which asserts that the quality of life, especially in relation to less street crime, was much better 20 years earlier. Pearson's analyses of *Punch* and other magazines and newspapers show in graphic detail that hooliganism and theft in the street accompanied by violence (what is now called 'mugging') were quite common in urban areas in nineteenth-century Britain.

Letters

Along with a life history, the analysis of letters played a central part in Thomas and Znaniecki's *The Polish Peasant in Europe and America*. For example, the authors were able to gain access to letters sent by emigrés to relatives in Poland, which they used to gain insight into the experiences of assimilation into American culture. The problem with the use of letters in social research is that they have a tendency not to be very focused, though where they are they can be a valuable source of unsolicited data. This is the case, for example, with letters written on a specific issue to newspapers, which can be used to identify differing and sometimes conflicting political viewpoints in relation to that issue.

Stories, essays and other writings

Researchers can make use of essays or other writings which are already in existence or can solicit such writings as part of their research design. For example, analyses of childrens' writings have been used to explore their experience of home, family and social relations (Steedman, 1982), whereas Cohen and Taylor's (1972) examination of the subjective experiences of imprisonment and strategies of psychological survival among long-term prisoners was in part founded on an analysis of essays and poems on topics suggested by Cohen and Taylor themselves. This strategy was consistent with the qualitative, naturalistic and discovery-based methodological approach, directed at uncovering the subjective experiences of prisoners, and it was also appropriate on practical grounds in so far as Cohen and Taylor gained access to the prison and to prisoners in their role as visiting, part-time lecturers. As such, they were in an ideal position to solicit essays and other writings for research purposes.

Official documents and records

A great many official documents and records on a wide range of topics are available for analysis. An important part of the activities of state relates to the production of official documents as, for instance, forerunners to legislation (as is the case with Green Papers and White Papers), as part of the regular review of activities of Departments of State or institutions under their control (e.g. reports of Select Committees of the House of Commons), or as part of the investigation of events or problems in the running of institutions (as is the case with some Royal Commissions). The discussion of critical analyses of documents in Section 4 will consider two such official documents: the Control Review Committee on Prisons (an example of a regular review) and the Woolf Inquiry into prison disturbances (an example of a one-off investigation of problems in one sector of state-controlled institutions). Official documents provide valuable data for the analysis of official definitions of what is defined as problematic, what is viewed as the explanation of the problem, and what is deemed to be the preferred solution. In this way, the analysis of such documents provides an important element in the critical analysis of texts.

Apart from documents at a societal or macro level, there are other official documents at an institutional or micro level which can be just as important to the disposal and destiny of individuals. These are organizational records which define what is, or is not, problematic about individuals, which put forward explanations for behaviour and actions and which record decisions relating to outcomes. Of course, such individual records are not necessarily separate from official documents operating at a societal level in so far as there is often a close interconnection between the formulation of concepts, explanations and solutions at one level and such formulation and application at another. Official records from a variety of settings have been examined. For example, Kitsuse and Cicourel (1963), working within what will later be described as an *interpretative* approach, analysed pupils' records to make assertions about the labels and stereotypes assigned by teachers, and about the consequences of these. In Section 4 we shall consider the writings of Anne Worrall (1990) who, working within what is subsequently described as the *critical* approach, examined the discourses of solicitors, magistrates, psychiatrists and probation officers, and the consequences these have for the disposal of women offenders.

There is one further type of document which is of particular interest to us in a course on research methods: namely, reports of social research findings and conclusions written by academics and other researchers (perhaps government-sponsored researchers). The position taken in this unit is that such reports should not be treated as objective, accurate statements of 'fact', but as documents which require examination and challenge in terms of what they define as problematic, the way in which such problems are operationalized, the forms of explanation which are put forward and the policy implications which flow from them. A critical analysis of particular research reports is important in instances where such reports hold a high profile and an influential position in the public domain. Audio-cassette 2 (which you will be asked to listen to in Section 4.6) will return once again to the reading concerning the Cambridge Study in Delinquent Development which you came across in Unit 9. Instead of subjecting it to a 'technical' evaluation (e.g. asking questions about sample size, response rates, levels of statistical significance), a 'critical' analysis, in the terms of Section 4, will be undertaken (e.g. asking questions about what is and is not seen as problematic, what is and is not seen as the explanation, and what is and is not seen as the preferred solution).

A typology of documents

Scott (1990) has produced a typology of documents based on two main criteria: authorship and access (see Table 1). Authorship refers to the origins of documents and under this heading he distinguishes 'personal' documents from 'official' ones (which have their source in bureaucracies). Official documents are further subdivided into 'state' and 'private' (i.e. non-state: for example, business annual reports and accounts). The second criterion, access, refers to the availability of documents to individuals other than the authors. 'Closed' documents are available only to a limited number of insiders, usually those who produce them; 'restricted' documents are available on an occasional basis provided permission has been granted; 'open-archival' documents are those documents which are stored in archives and are available to those who know of them and know how to access them; 'open-published' documents are the most accessible of all and are in general circulation.

Table 1   A classification of documents

		Authorship		
		Personal	Official	
			Private	State
Access	Closed	1	5	9
	Restricted	2	6	10
	Open-archival	3	7	11
	Open-published	4	8	12

(Source: Scott, 1990, p.14)

ACTIVITY I

Which documents do you think illustrate Types 1–12, using Scott's description shown in Table 1? Refer to the range of documents mentioned in this section and also to those discussed in Unit 13. Write down your list before consulting the answer at the end of this unit.

Such classifications can be useful in themselves. However, for Scott the usefulness of a classification based on the criteria he suggests is that it poses four key questions pertaining to the validity of particular documentary sources. Who has and has not authored a document, and the degree to which a document is accessible or withheld, influences its *authenticity* (whether it is original and genuine); its *credibility* (whether it is accurate); its *representativeness* (whether it is representative of the totality of documents of its class); and its *meaning* (what it is intended to say). This list encompasses most of the questions included in Section 5.3, 'Summary of some further questions to ask', in Unit 13. You should refresh your memory of these before moving on.

2.2 THE USE OF DOCUMENTS

ACTIVITY 2

Write a few notes on the ways in which you think documents could be used in research. Where possible, use examples from preceding parts of the course. To help prompt your thoughts, think about ways in which documents can be used:

(a) at different stages of research;

(b) in conjunction with other methods of research;

(c) as the sole source of data.

The literature search and evaluation is a vital preliminary to most social inquiry and within that, of course, documentary sources play a central part. The range of sources is not restricted to academic writings but can encompass the full spectrum outlined in the previous section. The literature review plays an important role in the early formulation of the general research problem, and in the further refinement of research questions, and may even be the source of specific hypotheses. Where documents give access to actors' concepts and perspectives, the development of theory to guide subsequent research can be 'grounded' in such concepts and perspectives. For example, an analysis of school records may show that teachers consistently use concepts such as 'duds', 'deadbeats', 'spurters' and 'high-fliers' to distinguish pupils. Such concepts can form the basis of theoretical concepts used in explanations of decision making by teachers and of subsequent effects on pupil careers. Where documents are used in formulation of problems, questions, hypotheses and theoretical developments, they are often referred to as 'sensitizing devices'.

With regard to research design, especially survey research design, a reading of relevant documents can give insights into how a population ought to be defined in terms of the significant groups or sub-groups to be included, and also into how the sample should be selected, perhaps in terms of the appropriate stratification factors to be used. Documents can also be used to suggest the topics to be covered in questionnaires, especially in terms of those topics which are most meaningful to the subjects themselves, and to help in the formulation of question wording in ways that are understandable to them. With regard to ethnographic research, the researcher will typically use secondary sources to gain a detailed knowledge of the type of social setting under consideration, the range of groups it includes and the potential problems of access.

There are occasions when documentary sources are used alongside other forms of data collection as a predetermined part of the research design. For example, in Unit 9 detailed reference was made to the Cambridge Study in Delinquent Development (Farrington, 1989), a longitudinal survey of young people, some of whom were to become offenders and others who were not. The survey was largely based on interviews with the young people, their families and teachers. However, it also used documentary sources in order to check the validity of data about

UNIT 21 CRITICAL ANALYSIS OF TEXT

offenders collected from self-report interviews. The use of one method to validate conclusions drawn from another method is known as *triangulation* (see, for example, Denzin, 1978), a term to which you were introduced in earlier units of this course.

Unit 9 also introduced ways in which documents can be used on their own in social inquiry. For example, it was noted that social surveys are sometimes assumed to apply exclusively to samples of individuals. However, other units can be sampled, including documents. The formal use of documents in this way is sometimes known as content analysis and will be introduced in the next section. Documents may also become the sole source of data. This can occur where there is no means of gaining access to respondents, even if this were desirable, or where respondents are dead. It is for the latter reason that documents play an important part in historical research.

A useful distinction emerges from the above examples, namely between documents as *resources* in research and documents as *objects* of research. Where documents assist in problem formulation, in research design decisions or to triangulate with other forms of data, they can be viewed as resources in research. Where documents represent the sole focus, they can be viewed as the objects of research. The emphasis in this unit is on the latter. This is especially the case with regard to critical analysis of text, in which documents are treated as objects of inquiry in their own right, especially in terms of their being mechanisms by which knowledge and power are applied.

3 TRADITIONS IN DOCUMENTARY ANALYSIS

This section, and Section 4 which follows, consider the ways in which three broad theoretical paradigms have each influenced the analysis of documents.

READING

You should now turn to Chapter 5, 'Traditions in documentary analysis' by Victor Jupp and Clive Norris, in the Reader. Read the section headed 'The origins of documentary analysis'. While reading, make notes on the following:

1   What is the importance of Thomas and Znaniecki's work?

2   What main theoretical and methodological strands can be detected in the development of documentary analysis?

Historically, the analysis of documents has played an important part in academic endeavour. However, Thomas and Znaniecki's work was influential in establishing documentary analysis within twentieth-century social science. They were concerned with aspects of Polish immigration into the USA, especially Chicago, during the 1920s. Their book *The Polish Peasant in Europe and America* is renowned for its use of personal and other documents. These included letters that emigrés sent back home, a major life history of Vladeck, a Polish peasant, materials from a newspaper established by Polish immigrants, official documents from agencies in Poland, and records and reports from social work agencies and courts in the USA.

With regard to the second question you were asked, three main strands in documentary analysis are discernible — the positivist, the interpretative and the critical. It is important to recognize that these represent very broad paradigms and include within them a number of sub-plots. Also, one should be wary of seeing positivist, interpretative and critical approaches as mutually exclusive, because they blur at the edges and so any given piece of documentary analysis cannot always be neatly pigeonholed as positivist, interpretative or critical: researchers take their influences from a number of different sources.

3.1 THE POSITIVIST AND INTERPRETATIVE USES OF DOCUMENTS

READING

At this point, you should read the sections entitled 'Positivism and documents' and 'The interpretative tradition and documents', in Chapter 5 of the Reader. While reading, make notes on the following:

1 What are the main features of the positivist use of documents?

2 What are the main features of the interpretative use of documents?

The positivist approach to documents — sometimes referred to as *content analysis* — is typified by Holsti (1969), who itemized five main features. These are that procedures should be *systematic* and *objective*, the analysis should have *generality*, it should be *quantitative* and it should focus on the *manifest content* of documents. Content analysts are interested in counting the number of times particular words or themes appear in a document — a newspaper, for example. They may also measure the number of column inches given to particular kinds of stories — crime stories as opposed to others, for example — or the size of headlines associated with types of stories. These procedures have led to the viewpoint that content analysis is a purely technical process:

> Once the initial categories are chosen, it is possible for techniques to be applied by assistants who have not been involved in the development of the theory and to be checked for technical objectivity by adherents of rival theoretical frameworks. The origin of the categories is assumed to be irrelevant to the formal validity of the method. It has even been argued that content analysis could be undertaken by an appropriately programmed computer, using index and data-base systems as alternatives to human researchers.
>
> (Scott, 1990, p.131)

Typically, research designs cluster around one or more of the following questions: What are the characteristics of the content? What inferences can be made about the causes and generation of content? What inferences can be made about the effects of communication? In emphasizing the manifest content of documents there is an assumption that the content unambiguously represents the meaning, and the latter is therefore treated neither as problematic nor as a prime focus of interest. This is what is meant by the Representational Model — the content *represents* the meaning.

By way of contrast, the interpretative approach places social meanings at the centre of any analysis; that is, meanings attributed to the contents of documents by producers and by audiences and the subsequent consequences for individuals and social groups. In doing this, the interpretative tradition is at odds with the positivist assumptions of a correspondence between intent, content and effect on different audiences and of the belief that there is a common universe of meanings uniting all relevant parties. What the interpretative tradition brings to the research agenda is a focus on the ways in which meanings are assigned both by authors and audiences and the subsequent consequences. The interpretative approach to documents is very close to the ethnographic tradition in social research.

4 CRITICAL SOCIAL RESEARCH

Harvey (1990) distinguishes critical social research as follows:

> Critical social research is underpinned by a critical–dialectical perspective which attempts to dig beneath the surface of historically specific oppressive social structures. This is contrasted with positivistic concerns to discover the factors that cause observed phenomena or to build grand theoretical edifices and with phenomenological attempts to interpret the meanings of social actors or attempt close analysis of symbolic processes.
>
> (Harvey, 1990, p.1)

This quotation reveals some of the differences between critical research and, on the one hand, positivism (which is often, but not exclusively, associated with quantitative research such as surveys, experimentation and content analysis) and, on the other hand, phenomenology which is roughly equivalent to what we have termed the interpretative tradition (and often, but not exclusively, associated with ethnographic research). The differences which are highlighted are as follows: first, positivism emphasizes explanations cast in causal terms whereas critical research does not; second, whilst both interpretative and critical perspectives are concerned with social meanings of, for example, contents of documents, the former places emphasis on how these are generated in small-scale interactions whereas the latter seeks to analyse them critically in terms of structural inequalities in society (e.g. class, race or gender inequalities).

Within the social sciences the critical tradition owes much to Marx or to reworkings of Marx by other writers. Critical research which is influenced by this source is concerned with social structural inequalities founded on class inequalities. The work of the American sociologist, C. Wright Mills, was influenced by the Marxist tradition but was less explicitly class based in directing its attention at bureaucratization in mass society and at the concentration of power in a power élite (see especially Mills, 1956). During the 1970s the critical tradition received impetus from the rise of black movements and from feminism. This led to the examination of structures founded on race and gender inequalities.

There are variations within the critical tradition. Nevertheless, a number of central assumptions is discernible. First, prevailing knowledge (e.g. that provided in official documents such as reports of Royal Commissions) is viewed as being structured by existing sets of social relations which constitute social structure. Second, this structure is seen as oppressive in so far as there is an unequal relation between groups within it and in so far as one or more groups exercise power over others. Third, the inequality, power and oppression are rooted in class, race or gender or some combination of these. Fourth, the aim of critical analysis is not to take prevailing knowledge for granted or to treat it as some 'truth', but to trace back such knowledge to structural inequalities at particular intersections in history. In doing so, it is considered important to examine the role of ideology in the maintenance of oppression and control and also the way in which social processes and social institutions operate to legitimate that which is treated as knowledge. Ultimately, the aim of critical research and analysis is to confront prevailing knowledge — and the structures which underpin it — by providing an alternative reading and understanding of it.

READING

You should now read Brian Fay's 'The elements of critical social science'. This is Chapter 4 in the Reader.

The reading by Fay epitomizes the central features of critical research as outlined above. However, in its emphasis on *emancipation* it goes one step further. For Fay it is not sufficient that critical research enlightens oppressed groups by providing an analysis of the root causes of such oppression. Such enlightenment should lead to emancipation: 'By offering this complex set of analyses to the relevant group at the appropriate time in the appropriate setting, a social theory can legitimately hope not only to explain a social order but to do so in such a way that this order is overthrown' (Fay, 1987, in Hammersley, 1993, p.36).

Deconstruction and reconstruction

The twin concepts of deconstruction and reconstruction are central to much critical research. Deconstruction is the process by which prevailing knowledge, or any construct within it, is broken down into its essential elements. This can involve the collection of empirical data and the examination of such data in relation to the abstract constructs which constitute knowledge. Reconstruction involves the rebuilding of a construct in terms of the oppressive social structural arrangements which underpin it and sustain it.

An example is required in order to illustrate what is otherwise an abstract set of prescriptions for analysis. We can take the construct 'housework', which can be deconstructed or broken down in terms of a set of activities and tasks which are viewed within prevailing knowledge as constituting its essence (washing dishes, ironing clothes, etc.). The process of reconstruction involves an examination of this construct in terms of wider structural arrangements, especially gender inequalities in society. It may also provide an analysis in terms of class (e.g. a study of working-class housewives) and class and race (e.g. a study of black working-class housewives). Such reconstruction views 'housework' not as a set of activities such as washing dishes, making beds and so forth, but as an exploitative relationship within a social structure with patterned inequalities and oppressions.

4.1 CRITICAL ANALYSIS OF DOCUMENTS

Critical analysis is explicitly theoretical. However, empirical work has been and is carried out, including social surveys, detailed interviews, social history research, participant observation and, of course, the analysis of documents. (For examples of the use of each of these in critical research see Harvey, 1990.) The contribution which the analysis of documents can make within the critical research tradition is indicated in the reading 'Traditions in documentary analysis'.

READING

You should now read the section entitled 'The critical tradition', in Chapter 5 in the Reader. While reading the extract ask yourself:

1. What are the main features of the critical tradition and how do they differ from positivism on the one hand and the interpretative approach on the other?

2. What questions might form the core of a research agenda organized around the critical analysis of documents?

The key features of the critical tradition can be highlighted by comparison with the features of positivism and the interpretative approach as outlined in Section 3. The critical tradition is critical both of positivism and of the interpretative tradition whilst agreeing with the latter about the relevance of the assignment of social meanings and subsequent consequences. However, further and more 'critical' concerns are added to the research agenda. These include a concern with analysis at a societal and social structural level; an emphasis on social conflict; an emphasis on power and control; an interest in ideology as a means by which existing social arrangements are legitimated; and a commitment to not taking for granted what is said. With specific reference to the analysis of documents, there is therefore an interest in the role of official, quasi-official and other documents, an emphasis on the role of such documents in social conflict and as mechanisms by which power is exercised, and an interest in documents as legitimating devices.

4.2 DISCOURSE ANALYSIS

An important development within the critical paradigm stems from the writings of the French social theorist Michel Foucault and relates to what is termed discourse analysis. The meaning of 'discourse' in social science has already been discussed in Section 2 in this unit, and earlier in the course in Unit 16.

READING

At this point you should turn once more to Chapter 5 in the Reader and read the sections entitled 'Discourse analysis' and 'Conclusion'. While reading, ask yourself the following questions:

1 What are the key assumptions of discourse analysis?

2 What is distinctive about the Foucauldian approach to discourse analysis?

3 What are the main elements of the research agenda which is suggested?

One key assumption is that discourse is social, which indicates that words and their meanings depend on where they are used and by whom, to whom. Consequently, their meaning can vary according to social and institutional settings and there is, therefore, no such thing as a universal discourse. Second, there can be different discourses which may be in conflict with one another. Third, as well as being in conflict, discourses may be viewed as being arranged in a hierarchy: the notions of conflict and of hierarchy link closely with the exercise of power. The concept of power is vital to discourse analysis via the theoretical connection between the production of discourses and the exercise of power. The two are very closely interwoven and, in some theoretical formulations, are viewed as one and the same.

The Foucauldian approach to discourse analysis is distinctive on a number of counts including the position that discourse and power are one and the same: 'Power produces knowledge, they imply one another: a site where power is exercised is also a place at which knowledge is produced' (Smart, 1989, p.65). What is more, Foucault's position is that there is not one focus of knowledge and power (e.g. the state) but several:

> His viewpoint is that strategies of power and social regulation are pervasive and that the state is only one of several points of control. This is an important divergence from Marxist analysis. For Foucault there are many semi-autonomous realms in society, where the state has little influence, but where power and control is exercised. In this way Foucault's notion of the pervasiveness of loci of regulation and control encourages research about discourses in a range of institutional settings.
>
> (Jupp and Norris, 1993, in Hammersley, 1993, p.49)

The ways in which research may be carried out in such settings are laid out in the 'research agenda' in the conclusion to the chapter. The 'agenda' brings together questions which typically would be asked in a critical analysis of documents, especially with reference to discourse analysis. It is unlikely that any given analysis will deal with all these questions; rather, it will tend to focus on some to the exclusion of others.

Critical analysis, and discourse analysis in particular, has a tendency towards being theoretical. It is appropriate, especially in a course concerned with social research methods, to consider how an abstract set of ideas and concepts can be converted into a programme for research. This will be done in the following sections via a number of case studies, each of which uses different types of documents and represents a different selection of research questions, from the above agenda, with which to address the documents.

The first case study is of a fictitious research proposal to carry out discourse analysis on what — using Scott's typology in Section 2.1 — can be called 'state' documents which are 'open-published'; that is, they are in general circulation. This case study is especially useful because it shows how a particular theoretical system can be turned into a programme of research. The second case study shows the end product of a critical analysis of an open state document. It illustrates the conclusion which one social scientist, Mike Fitzgerald, reached after a critical 'reading' of a report on prisons. The third case study is based on institutional records and transcripts of detailed interviews with professionals in the criminal justice system to examine decision making regarding the disposal of women offenders. The final case study involves a different form of document, a report of survey findings produced by social researchers. This case study illustrates the difference between a critical analysis of text and a 'technical' evaluation of research design and the findings derived from it. This case study can be found on Audio-cassette 2.

4.3 CASE STUDY 1: A PROPOSAL FOR CRITICAL ANALYSIS

READING

You should now read the following example of a research proposal based on critical analysis of a text. Write notes on these questions:

1. Which, if any, of the research questions included in the agenda at the end of Chapter 5 in the Reader are represented in the proposal?

2. What method of inquiry is advocated and how does it differ from positivist content analysis?

Official analyses of problems in prisons

Introduction

The transformation of a sequence of events into what becomes defined as a deep-seated 'social problem' is often marked by the setting up of a public inquiry. The theoretical analyses and moral perspective of such inquiries play a large part in determining public perception of 'normality' and 'dangerousness'. In 1990 serious rioting took place in Strangeways Prison, Manchester. The government of the day commissioned Lord Justice Woolf to conduct inquiries into the rioting. Woolf decided to adopt a broad interpretation of his terms of reference to address wider issues which the disturbances raised (e.g. physical conditions in prisons, the use of local prisons to keep individuals on remand, the extent of overcrowding). The Report of the Woolf Commission was published in 1991 (Woolf, 1991).

Research questions

Two sets of important questions can be asked about the Woolf Report, or, indeed, any other such official report. First, we can try to ascertain the nature of the official discourse it represents:

- How does Woolf define the *problems* of our prisons in the 1990s?
- What range of *explanations* does he consider?
- What does he propose as the *control solution*?

Second, and more generally, we could investigate the role of such public 'voices' as Woolf's, perhaps by comparing the Report with other official or quasi-official reports. For example, in relation to crime and criminal justice we could undertake 'readings' of the Scarman Report on the Brixton disorders of 1981 (Scarman, 1981) or of the Taylor Report on the Hillsborough disaster (Taylor, 1990). However, we need not restrict ourselves to this area of concern. Instead, we can investigate a wide range of official reports (e.g. on health, education and housing). The important questions to ask are:

- What is the *audience* addressed by these official reports and for whom do they speak?
- What *influence* do reports of this kind have on what happens in agencies of social control?

Theoretical frameworks

Much of the interest today in official discourses stems from the influence of Michel Foucault on social science. Foucault envisages society not as something 'out there' which causes, and is in turn reacted upon by, certain kinds of knowledge or social policy. Rather, 'society' comprises an array of *discourses* which exhibit and produce moral norms, theoretical explanations and techniques of social control. These three aspects of social regulation are, in Foucault's view, quite inseparable. So, the first three research questions listed aim to try to establish the various components of official discourse about problems in prisons and the overall moral climate such discourse creates.

The second set of questions gets us to think about who is represented in public discourse of this kind. On whose behalf does Woolf speak — the liberal professions? the ruling class? the Establishment? And whom is he addressing — the moral majority? the British public? the respectable white male citizen? It is important to recognize here that, for Foucault, these 'subjects', on both sides, are not concrete individuals or groups existing *outside* the field of the discourse itself. Rather, they are 'ideal' positions which are produced in and through such discourses, serving as powerful moral regulators. The last questions further reflect Foucault's view that official discourse is only *one* type amongst others, and that the social priorities established in any given discourse may well be undercut or qualified by those established in other discourses (such as those of the media or the police).

Methods of inquiry

This project involved 'reading' and reflecting upon Woolf and similar official reports, looking closely at the way in which language is used, and at the values involved, so as to produce the typical 'subject' of the discourse. Reports embody certain types of theory or knowledge — which may be embodied in policy and institutions — about what or who is the problem, about what is the explanation and about what is the 'correct' solution. Considerations of power are deeply embedded in such theory and knowledge. The purpose of 'reading' is to apprehend such theory, knowledge and power. This type of approach does not accept a distinction between the 'theoretical' and the 'empirical' modes of investigation.

The research proposal has the analysis of the report of the Woolf Inquiry at its centre. In doing so, it enlists theoretical ideas from Foucault, particularly the viewpoint that society comprises an array of discourses which express and produce moral norms defining what are 'right' explanations and techniques of control. The report of the Woolf Inquiry is one such official discourse relating to prisons. It provided official definitions of what is wrong with our prisons, why these problems exist and how they should be solved. (The precise recommendations are not reproduced here. For a useful summary and commentary consult Sparks, 1992.) The theoretical ideas derived from Foucault generate research questions to be asked of the Report at two levels. First of all, one set of questions is asked of the document itself. These questions are concerned with what is defined as problematic (and, by implication, what is not defined as problematic); the explanations or theories that are provided (and, by implication, the explanations that are omitted or rejected); the solutions that are offered (and, by implication, the solutions that are rejected). These are typical of questions 5 and 6 of the research agenda outlined in the conclusion to Chapter 5 in the Reader.

A second set of questions relates not to the document itself but to the 'subjects' on either side, asking on whose behalf the report speaks and to whom it speaks. These are close to questions 3 and 4 in the research agenda. Note that, in contrast to the interpretative approach outlined earlier in this unit, the focus in the approach advocated in this proposal is not upon the actual person who wrote the report, nor is it upon the actual people who read it. Rather, it is upon 'ideal' positions which are produced in and through such discourses, serving as powerful regulators.

With regard to methods of inquiry, the position adopted is in complete contrast to that of positivist content analyses. There is no reference to formal protocol of categorization, coding and counting of words, themes, headlines or column inches. Rather, the project involves 'reading' and 'reflecting' and is founded upon an approach that does not accept that there are two separate yet interrelated activities of theorizing and empirical research carried out by two different kinds of people: theorists and research technicians.

4.4 CASE STUDY 2: CRITICAL ANALYSIS OF A PUBLIC DOCUMENT

READING

You should now read 'The telephone rings: long-term imprisonment', by Mike Fitzgerald, in Offprints Booklet 4. The article is a critical analysis of a public document about prisons. In reading it you do not need to know about specialist issues in penology; rather, you should focus on the methodological approach used by Fitzgerald. In particular, write notes on the following:

1 What *kinds* of documents is Fitzgerald concerned with? Refer back to Scott's typology of documents outlined in Section 2.1.

2 What *aspects* of the documents is he concerned with? In particular, focus on definitions of what is seen as problematic in the documents, preferred solutions to these problems and implied theory of management.

Fitzgerald focuses on a number of official reviews, inquiries and policy papers that have followed disorders in prisons, with a view to uncovering the principles of penal policy that underpin their recommendations. In terms of the typology outlined earlier, the documents can be classified as official–state–open-published.

In his consideration of the Report of the Control Review Committee, Fitzgerald focuses on three main areas that make up what he calls the 'general orientation' of the Report. This general orientation, and its three sub-areas, constitute the object of analysis. First, he is concerned with the concepts that the Committee employs to define that which it sees as problematic, and he then goes on to deconstruct some of these concepts to see how they themselves are defined. For example, he notes that 'control' is central to the Committee's conceptualization and also that control is defined in terms of the control of the prisoners themselves, whereas other reports have sought to conceptualize this in terms of problems in the Prison Service. In short, this form of analysis asks why certain kinds of concepts, defined in certain ways, are placed on the public agenda.

Second, he is concerned with the kinds of solutions that emerge from the Committee's thinking. As he points out, such solutions are largely in terms of new prison designs and not in other terms, such as improving prisoner–staff relations. The preferred solution does not stand in isolation but flows directly from the way in which the Committee conceptualizes what is seen as being problematic in the prison system.

Third, Fitzgerald analyses the implicit theory of management that underpins both the conceptualization of the problem and the preferred solution and its implementation. As he argues, he is not against management *per se* but questions the rigid hierarchical theory of management that dominates the thinking of the Committee.

At this point it is appropriate to summarize some of the key features of the critical approach to documents in the light of Fitzgerald's analysis of the Report of the Control Review Committee.

- First, the sources of data are often, but not always, official texts which are important at a macro level in so far as they put forward conceptualizations regarding, in this case, the prison system, although they could refer to any other element of the social system.

- Second, the method does not exhibit the formal protocols of quantitative content analysis (e.g. categorizing, coding, counting), but is a critical reading of texts aimed at uncovering how problems are defined, what explanations are put forward and what is seen as the preferred solution. It also seeks to bring to the surface that which is rejected in the text and that which does not even appear — what is *not* seen as problematic, what explanations are not considered, and what are not the preferred solutions. In other words, the analysis is concerned with how official documents frame the public agenda.

- Third, Fitzgerald is not solely concerned with analysing the definitions, explanations and solutions put forward in official documents, but seeks to challenge them and suggests alternative proposals and viewpoints. In this sense, the methodological approach is not exclusively a critical reading of the text, but is also a challenge to the text.

- Fourth, note that the paper is solely concerned with the 'communication'; that is, with the text. It could have gone beyond this by examining the 'senders' and the 'recipients'. Had it done so it would not have been concerned with the identity of individual authors or with the meanings they bring to the text as someone from the interpretative tradition would be, but with the section of society for whom the document speaks, and with the consequences for the prison system and its inhabitants.

- Finally, unlike the preceding research proposal given in Section 4.3, Fitzgerald does not make explicit reference to discourse analysis or to Foucauldian theory in general. There are similarities in approach, although there are also differences. This is not the place to go into the fine details of different theoretical and methodological positions. It is sufficient to note that Fitzgerald's paper exemplifies the critical approach to documents as epitomized in the research agenda at the end of Chapter 5 in the Reader, an agenda which in good part was influenced by the work of Michel Foucault.

4.5 CASE STUDY 3: CRITICAL ANALYSIS OF DECISION MAKING

The next reading, also within the critical tradition, is slightly different from the preceding two case studies in so far as it is not concerned with macro state-originated documents. Rather, it involves transcripts of detailed interviews with 'experts' within the criminal justice system and institutional records. What is more, it is not solely concerned with one discourse, namely that represented in official state reports on prisons, but with a multiplicity of interacting discourses which have consequences for the decisions made regarding women who offend.

READING

You should now read the three short extracts from Anne Worrall's *Offending Women* which you will find in Offprints Booklet 4. The first extract outlines the theoretical and methodological position of the author; the second details the research methods which were used; the third summarizes the main conclusion. You might find it helpful to 'skim-read' in the first instance, followed by more detailed study. Write notes on the following:

1 What methodological approach is preferred?

2 What is the relationship between power and knowledge?

3 What is the relationship between discourse and practice?

4 What are the implications of discourse analysis for methodology?

5 How was the research carried out in practice?

6 What discourses lay claim to knowledge about women offenders and are therefore important in relation to the disposal of such offenders?

The position taken by Worrall eschews social science which, on the one hand, is concerned with the search for universal properties and causes and, on the other hand, is solely concerned with social meanings. She is not interested in questions of what is the 'truth', but rather with 'the relationship between those who claim to know the "truth" and those about whom they claim to know it' (Worrall, 1990, p.6). In turn, this relates to the question, 'What is it that endows certain individuals to have such knowledge and to apply it?'. These are the hallmarks of critical analyses in general and of discourse analysis in particular.

The relationship between power and knowledge is vital to such analyses. Worrall's viewpoint is that knowledge does not of itself give power. Rather, those who have power have the authority to know. In this context such people are magistrates, probation officers, solicitors and psychiatrists. Power is not reducible to one source, class (as Marxist analyses would have it), but exists in all social relations. In this case, it exists in the relations between women offenders and those who make decisions about them, and also in the relations between such decision makers themselves. Within this analysis the exercise of power is not the naked oppression of one group by another but the production and subtle application of coherent 'knowledge' about other individuals which has consequences for what happens to these individuals (e.g. Social Inquiry Reports, written by probation officers about offenders, which can influence decisions taken about such offenders). This is discourse as discussed at the beginning of Section 2.

Discourses have implications for practice in terms of programmes, technologies and strategies: that is, coherent sets of explanation and solutions, ways of implementing these solutions and strategies of intervention. The earlier discussion of discourse analysis (in Section 4.2) indicated that there can be differing and competing discourses.

In this respect, Worrall suggests that the power of the offender lies in the ability to resist, and even refuse, the coherent and homogeneous discourse of 'experts': 'By demonstrating the existence of heterogeneity and contradiction, the speaking subject is helping to keep open the space within which knowledge is produced' (Worrall, 1990, p.10). In the main, however, women offenders remain markedly non-resistant and 'muted'.

The methodological approach is one of a case study of detailed interviews with magistrates, probation officers, psychiatrists and solicitors and of institutional records and reports. It has no claims to randomness or representativeness (as, for instance, a social survey would) and it seeks to generalize via theorizing rather than by reference to probability theory (again, as a survey would): 'The adoption of this particular mode of theorizing womens' experiences calls for a method of research which rejects notions of generalizability through probability in favour of generalization through theoretical production' (ibid., p.12). As with the first case study, we found rejection of the viewpoint that there are two distinct activities, theorizing and empirical inquiry.

The main conclusion of Worrall's work is that women are 'muted' within the criminal justice system by being subject to the multiple discourses of the 'experts' who are authorized to present coherent knowledge concerning problems, explanations and solutions and who deny legitimacy to the discourses of the women themselves. Worrall's analysis involves deconstructing the discourses of the 'experts'. Despite the power and authority of such discourses, offenders develop means of resisting them by exploiting construction within them: 'Yet, while much of the women's resistance is individualistic, inconsistent and, in some, self-destructive, it has the important effect of undermining the authority of official discourses and keeping open the possibility of the creation of new knowledge about them — both as women and as law-breakers' (ibid., p.163).

The contribution which this case study makes to the discussion of critical analysis is that, in comparison with the other examples, it shows that there can be a multiplicity of discourses, that these can operate in subtle ways, that there can be resistances to prevailing discourses, and that outcomes have a good deal to do with the positions of particular discourses in the hierarchy of legitimacy and authority.

4.6 CASE STUDY 4: CRITICAL ANALYSIS OF A RESEARCH REPORT

ACTIVITY 3

You should now listen to Audio-cassette 2, Side 2. Before doing so, though, you should read the appropriate notes in Section 2.3 of the Audio-Visual Handbook and the article by David Farrington, 'The origins of crime: the Cambridge Study in Delinquent Development', in Offprints Booklet 2, which you read in conjunction with Unit 9.

5 CONCLUSION

This unit has been concerned with the use of documents in social science research. Such documents include life histories, letters, diaries, essays, institutional memoranda, and public pronouncements such as Reports of Royal Commissions. They can also include reports of academic and policy-related research. The types of documents illustrated have been distinguished according to their authorship and also according to the degree to which they are accessible to researchers. A classification based upon these two criteria encourages us to ask questions pertaining to the validity of particular documentary sources; for example, whether a document is authentic, whether it is accurate, whether it is representative of other documents of its type and what is the intended meaning.

Three broad approaches to the use of documents have been outlined: the positivist, the interpretative and the critical. The emphasis in this unit has been on the critical approach to the use of documents as objects of inquiry (as opposed to resources in inquiry). The reason for this is that both positivist and interpretative approaches have been reflected elsewhere in the course (e.g. in the consideration of survey research and ethnographic research, respectively). Critical research is distinguished by questions which are asked of documents, especially questions about what does — and does not — constitute accepted 'knowledge' and with what consequences. By way of conclusion, three points are worthy of emphasis. First, as with positivist and interpretative approaches, critical analysis is used in a very broad sense within which there are different strands. For example, an approach influenced by Marxism places emphasis on the way in which documents reflect class oppression in society, whereas Foucauldian discourse analysis views power as operating at different levels and in different sectors of society and also does not reduce power to one source, namely class relations. Second, the unit (and its associated readings) may give the impression that there has been an historical unilinear development from positivist content analysis through interpretative analysis of documents to contemporary critical analysis. There is an element of truth in this in so far as, for example, interpretative approaches of the 1970s developed as a reaction to earlier positivism, and critical analyses of the 1980s responded to what were seen as shortcomings (e.g. insufficient attention paid to power) in interpretative approaches. Nevertheless, it should be recognized that all three approaches continue to exist alongside one another and to play their part in contemporary analysis of documents. Despite the emphasis of this unit, it would be wrong to assume that all documentary analysis is critical analysis. Finally, it would also be wrong to assume that critical research is solely concerned with documentary sources. As Harvey (1990) has illustrated, critical research encompasses a wide range of methods of research (e.g. interviews, surveys, observations) and forms of data (e.g. quantitative and qualitative, primary and secondary, contemporary and historical).

ANSWER TO ACTIVITY

ACTIVITY 1

Given below is a summary of the examples provided by Scott (1990) of the types of documents in his classification:

Type 1 Personal letters and diaries.

Type 2 Documents of a long-established land-owning family held in a private archive.

Type 3 Personal documents of such families deposited in a public archive for general use.

Type 4 Diaries of politicians written for subsequent publication.

Type 5 Confidential organizational memoranda.

Type 6 Company accounts and records held in their own offices.

Type 7 The governmental archive of business documents held at the companies Registration Office.

Type 8 Accounts of companies quoted on the Stock Exchange which, by law, must be published.

Type 9 State documents covered by the Official Secrets Act.

Type 10 Papers held in the Royal Archive which may be consulted if permission of the Sovereign is gained.

Type 11 Government papers classified as 'open', such as those held in the Public Record Office.

Type 12 State documents which are published, such as Annual Reports of Departments of State (e.g. Home Office).

REFERENCES

Allport, G.W. (1942) *The Use of Personal Documents in Psychological Science*, Social Science Research Council, Bulletin No. 49.

Boyle, J. (1984) *The Pain of Confinement*, London, Pan.

Cohen, S. (1972) *Folk Devils and Moral Panics*, London, Paladin.

Cohen, S. and Taylor, L. (1972) *Psychological Survival: The Experience of Long-Term Imprisonment*, Harmondsworth, Penguin.

Denzin, N. (1978) *The Research Act: A Theoretical Introduction to Sociological Methods*, 2nd edn, New York, McGraw-Hill.

Farrington, D. (1989) 'The origins of crime: the Cambridge Study in Delinquent Development', *Research Bulletin*, Home Office Research and Planning Unit, no. 27, pp.29–32 (reproduced in Offprints Booklet 2).

Fay, B. (1987) 'The elements of a critical social science', in Hammersley, M. (ed.) (1993) (DEH313 Reader).

Fitzgerald, M. (1987) 'The telephone rings: long-term imprisonment'; in Bottoms, A. and Light, L. (eds) *Problems of Long-Term Imprisonment*, Aldershot, Gower (reproduced in Offprints Booklet 4).

Hall, S., Critcher, C., Jefferson, T., Clarke, J. and Roberts, B. (1978) *Policing the Crisis: Mugging, the State and Law and Order*, London, Macmillan.

Hammersley, M. (ed.) (1993) *Social Research: Philosophy, Politics and Practice*, London, Sage (DEH313 Reader).

Harvey, L. (1990) *Critical Social Research*, London, Unwin Hyman.

Holsti, O.R. (1969) *Content Analysis for the Social Sciences and Humanities*, Reading, MA, Addison-Wesley.

Jupp, V. and Norris, C. (1993) 'Traditions in documentary analysis', in Hammersley, M. (ed.) (1993) (DEH313 Reader).

Kitsuse, J. and Cicourel, A.V. (1963) 'A note on the use of official statistics', *Social Problems*, vol. II, no. 2, pp.328–38.

Lewis, O. (1959) *Five Families*, New York, Basic Books.

Luria, A.R. (1972) *The Man with a Shattered World: The History of a Brain Wound*, New York, Basic Books.

Mills, C.W. (1956) *The Power Elite*, New York, Oxford University Press.

Pearson, G. (1983) *Hooligan: A History of Respectable Fears*, London, Macmillan.

Punch, M. (1985) *Conduct Unbecoming*, London, Tavistock.

Scarman, L.G. (1981) *The Brixton Disorders, April 10–12, 1981, Report of an Inquiry*, Home Office, Cmnd 8427, London, HMSO.

Scott, J. (1990) *A Matter of Record*, Cambridge, Polity.

Shaw, C. (1930) *The Jack Roller*, Chicago, IL, University of Chicago Press.

Smart, B. (1989) 'On discipline and social regulation: a review of Foucault's genealogical analysis', in Garland, D. and Young, P. (eds) *The Power to Punish*, London, Gower.

Sparks, R. (1992) 'The Prison Service as an organisation: 1979–91', Section A2 of *D803 Doing Prison Research*, Milton Keynes, Open University.

Steedman, C. (1982) *The Tidy House: Little Girls Writing*, London, Virago.

Taylor, Lord Justice P. (1990) *The Hillsborough Stadium Disaster, 15 April 1989, Inquiry by the Rt Hon. Lord Justice Taylor, Final Report*, Home Office, London, HMSO.

Thomas, W.I. and Znaniecki, F. (1958) *The Polish Peasant in Europe and America*, New York, Dover Publications (first published 1918–20).

Webb, E.J., Campbell, D.T., Schwartz, R.D. and Sechrest, L. (1966) *Unobtrusive Measures; Non-Reactive Research in Social Sciences*, Chicago, IL, Rand McNally.

Woolf, Lord Justice H.K. (1991) *Prison Disturbances April 1990, Report of an Inquiry by the Rt Hon. Lord Justice Woolf (Parts 1 and 2) and His Honour Judge Stephen Tumim (Part 2)*, Home Office, Cmnd 1456, London, HMSO.

Worrall, A. (1990) *Offending Women*, London, Routledge.

ACKNOWLEDGEMENT

Grateful acknowledgement is made to the following source for permission to reproduce material in this unit:

TABLE

Table 1: Scott, J. (1990) *A Matter of Record*, Polity Press.